LIVE A
Beautiful Life
with
LUPUS

Habits and Rituals for Thriving
with an Autoimmune Disease—
Body, Mind, and Spirit

OLIVIA DAVENPORT

CABIN CREEK PUBLISHING
RENO, NV

Publisher's Cataloging-in-Publication Data
provided by Five Rainbows Services

Davenport, Olivia.
  Live a beautiful life with lupus : habits and rituals for
thriving with an autoimmune disease : body, mind, and
spirit / Olivia Davenport.
    pages cm
  Includes bibliographical references.
  ISBN: 978-0-9967498-4-8 (pbk.)
  ISBN: 978-0-9967498-3-1 (e-book)
  1. Systemic lupus erythematosus—Patients—Life skills
guides. 2. Autoimmune diseases—Popular works. 3.
Holistic medicine. 4. Mind and body. 5. Self-care, Health.
I. Title.
RC924.5.L85 D37 2015
616.7`72—dc23
                                2015953189

Cover background image and flower motifs in book: Elenarts/iStock by Getty Images

Dedication

To my family:

Your support comforts me.
Your patience inspires me.
Your love sustains me.
From the deepest part of my soul,
I thank you.

Disclaimer of Warranty/Limit of Liability

Table of Contents

Introduction

I didn't set out to write a book about living with Lupus. My only intention in the beginning was to start a blog, which I did, based on the encouragement of a dear friend from journalism school. Thank you, Jeanne. My blog is called LupusDiary.com, and it's where I share how I live my life with an unpredictable autoimmune disease known as Lupus.

Jeanne was frank with me when she said that it would be a shame not to share my experiences after all these years, especially given the fact that in journalism school, we were trained to tell the stories that impact our world. While not necessarily newsworthy, the stories and events of my life with Lupus could be fodder for a made-for-TV movie, complete with crazy-life comedy juxtaposed with terrifying hospital scenes for dramatic effect.

So, I considered her suggestion and realized that I actually do have much to say. It was during that process of sorting my thoughts and reflecting on all that has happened over the last two decades, pre- and post- Lupus diagnosis, that I realized the need to share more than just the snippets of life that I write about on the blog. I felt the need to share what has now become a foundational part of who I am and how I choose to live—not as a victim of Lupus, but as someone who lives a beautiful life *with* Lupus.

I was diagnosed with Systemic Lupus Erythematosus (SLE or Lupus) in 2012, after suffering with episodes of illness—from mild to life threatening—since the birth of my son in 1991.

After so many years without knowing or understanding why I was sick and without having a label for what was wrong, I often found myself faced with two choices: either I could lie down and wait for death, being negative and unhappy about the hand that life had dealt me over and *over* again; or, I could find ways to adapt my life so that I could live as happily as possible.

Truth be told, as the mother of a bright-eyed baby boy who relied on me for everything, I really didn't have a choice early on. Once his father and I divorced when our son was just three years old, I had to make a life for us where we could both be happy and where he could grow up with the best that I could give him.

By trial and error, and lots of prayer and meditation, I found myself adapting to a life filled with uncertainty—not knowing if or when my next episode would strike. These episodes ranged from strange, random infections, debilitating headaches, and immobilizing arthritic pain to multiple, life-threatening complications with my heart and lungs, requiring repeated hospital stays and outpatient procedures.

With each hospitalization and prolonged absence from work, which ultimately led to my early retirement, I would find myself evaluating and re-evaluating what I must do to minimize the possibility of an episode happening again.

All along, I had no idea that these episodes would all be attributed to Lupus. All I knew was that I had to find a way to thrive despite whatever was going on—if not for myself, then for my young son.

With this book, my goal is to help those living with Lupus adapt to a life of uncertainty by understanding the disease and its impacts in order to work with their Lupus-altered body, mind, and spirit to achieve balance and harmony. For those of you who are new to Lupus as well as those who have lived with Lupus for many years, I hope the ideas and advice in this book will help you take a fresh look at how you're living your life while managing the disease. The book is divided into three parts, as follows:

Part I: What Does It Mean to Live a Beautiful Life? In this section, I discuss the concept of living a life of beauty and how it remains an elusive goal for even the healthiest of people. And, even though that definition varies from person to person, I'll explain how a holistic body-mind-spirit approach to overall health helps us get closer to that goal of living beautifully.

Part II: What Does It Mean to Live with Lupus? Here, I explain what it is to live with Lupus by defining the disease itself, separating fact from fiction, and going into detail about how Lupus affects each dimension of our being—the body, the mind, and the spirit.

Part III: It's Possible to Live a Beautiful Life with Lupus. In this section, I offer some hope that living a beautiful life and living with Lupus are not mutually exclusive. You can do both and prosper. It takes a bit of planning and working systematically through a framework of rituals and habits designed to soothe the Lupus body, strengthen the Lupus mind, and nurture the Lupus spirit.

Sure, it takes a bit of work, mostly a new awareness, a shift in perspective, and a commitment to make changes for your own well-being, but it can be done. I'm living proof, and I want to help you.

Love,

Olivia

P.S.—For more about me, and how I'm working to live a beautiful life with Lupus, please visit my websites at *www.lupusdiary.com* and *www.liveabeautifullifewithlupus.com*.

PART I:
What Does It Mean
to Live a Beautiful Life?

Chapter I:
The Concept of a Beautiful Life

"The longer I live, the more beautiful life becomes."
~Frank Lloyd Wright

What does it mean to live a beautiful life? If you posed that question to 10 people, you would likely get 10 different answers. Most answers would be along the lines of being happy, healthy, having all one's needs met, feeling satisfied with work or profession, enjoying wealth, peace at home and around the world.

The interesting thing is that each person would be right. Just like the concept of beauty itself, the meaning of living a beautiful life is truly personal and different for everyone. As British author Mary Wolfe Hungerford wrote in her novel, *Molly Bawn*, "Beauty is in the eye of the beholder."

Merriam-Webster defines beauty this way: "The quality or aggregate of qualities in a person or thing that gives pleasure to the senses or pleasurably exalts the mind or spirit."[1]

Another official definition of beauty comes from dictionary. com, where it is defined as: "The quality present in a thing or person that gives intense pleasure or deep satisfaction to the mind, whether arising from sensory manifestations (as shape, color, sound, etc.), a meaningful design or pattern, or something else (as a personality in which high spiritual qualities are manifest)."[2] So, basically, whatever gives you pleasure and satisfaction that you can see, feel, hear, taste, and/or smell—that's a thing or person of beauty. When we live our lives experiencing people, places, and things that give us that deep satisfaction—whatever those things may be—we're living a beautiful life.

Simple enough, right? Well, if it's so simple, then why do so many of us admit that we haven't gotten to the point where our lives are beautiful?

Despite living in one of the most prosperous countries in the world, Americans are increasingly unhappy, according to a 2014 poll conducted by two research groups—Anderson Robbins Research and Shaw and Company Research. The percentage of happy Americans, the poll indicates, has decreased from 68 percent in 2001, to 56 percent in 2009, to a low of 53 percent in 2014.[3]

The reasons vary, obviously, but at the top of the list are lack of job satisfaction and security, a difficult family or marriage situation, stagnant income and wages, high stress levels, the desire to "keep up with the Joneses," lack of sleep, and last but certainly not least, poor health.[4]

Many of these barriers to happiness are under our control. With enough determination, they can be overcome in order to succeed in making the changes necessary to find the beauty in life that so often eludes us. With specific work on key areas of our lives—the body, mind, and spirit—a renewed sense of motivation can uplift us enough to do whatever it takes to create our own version of a beautiful life.

But what about when you have constant illness in the form of a debilitating, chronic disease that has taken over your life? What happens when your physical body becomes the major hurdle to overcome, an unexpected barrier to success?

To live a beautiful life while living with a chronic illness takes a little more than the will to overcome. It takes the application of a framework, or a systematic approach, that will help you understand how the limitations of your body affect your mind and your overall spirit.

Viewing the body, mind, and spirit as a system of interdependent dimensions of our lives, we will see how important it is to manage each one, especially when living with a chronic illness, specifically Lupus.

Chapter 2:
Living Holistically—Body, Mind, and Spirit

"The part can never be well unless the whole is well."

~Plato

The body-mind-spirit philosophy represents the holistic view of who you are within the three dimensions of your being. It's the synergistic idea that the whole is greater when the sum of its individual parts work together.[5] When the three are in balance or not deficient in any way, life is wonderful. Your body functions well; your mind is clear, sharp, and emotionally healthy; and your spiritual connection to your sacred belief in something larger than yourself gives meaning to your life. All parts work together, holistically, to move you forward.

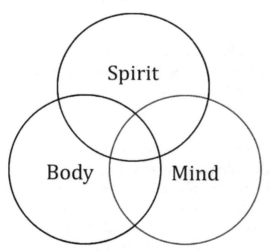

Figure 1: Body, Mind, and Spirit

Living holistically this way requires taking an objective look at each dimension to gain awareness. Only then will we be able to see where we can successfully improve, adjust, and adapt our circumstances as needed.

The Body

The body, the physical aspect of our being, is an amazing and miraculous machine of DNA, proteins, cells, neurons, and organ systems that work together to keep our hearts beating and pumping blood through 60,000 miles of blood vessels;[6] keep our lungs oxygenating our tissues; grow our hair and nails; digest food; eliminate waste; and fight off disease. Very simply put.

To operate efficiently, our bodies must be nurtured by the foods we eat, the amount of water we drink, along with a consistent amount of movement and exercise. When we fail to meet these basic needs, our bodies operate in a less-than-ideal state, due to poor nutrition, dehydration, or a sedentary lifestyle. This state can lead to disease, especially if the body is already predisposed genetically to certain illnesses, such as cancer, diabetes, and autoimmune diseases, like Lupus.

The Mind

The mind describes that inexplicable, unquantifiable dimension of our being that processes our environment—the sights, sounds, smells, tastes, and touch—and interprets it, giving meaning based on our own historical perceptions, experiences, and memories.

In much the same way as the body, the mind—this mental and emotional part of oneself—must be nurtured as well. Positive thinking, remaining open to learning, and the ability to adapt to life's unpredictability all contribute to a healthy mind.

When the mind is in a state of imbalance, due to negative thinking, anxiety, abnormal brain chemistry, and stress, it can have a detrimental effect on the body, causing physical manifestations, such as chest pain, a racing heart, headaches, upset stomach, aches, pains, tense muscles, insomnia...you get the picture. This also has a negative impact on the spiritual self by closing us off to the possibilities of connecting spiritually because we're too busy concentrating on and dealing with the battle going on in our own minds and bodies.

The Spirit

Spirit represents the life-giving, energizing force within a person that connects us to something larger than we are; something amorphous, invisible, but nevertheless present.[7]

Our spirit dimension is often where we transcend body and mind to "find meaning, hope, comfort, and inner peace" in our lives.[8]

Nurturing this dimension of our being comes in the form of meditation, prayer, service to our fellow humans, faithful religious practices, yoga, and an endless list of activities based on traditions, cultures and sacred beliefs. For some, spirituality encompasses religion, and for others it's a stand-alone concept with no attachment or affiliation to a religion or religious practice.[9] For purposes of this book, spirit and spirituality are referred to in the broadest sense.

When the spirit is in crisis or distress—when people are not able to connect with this force for one reason or another—the negativity in their lives is magnified. They feel hopelessness, a lack of meaning, disheartened, and inner turmoil. Often spiritual distress is the result of a direct conflict between their beliefs and what is actually happening in their lives.[10]

Oh, To Be Holistically Centered

So, we see that the body, mind, and spirit must each be nurtured and developed in such a way as to assist the whole human being in operating efficiently and progressively. We understand that each of the three is dependent on and affected by the other two. Ideally, your body, mind, and spirit work together to maximize your positive energy and overall well-being and to minimize stress, negative energy, and illness.

The point where the body, mind, and spirit overlap to create a balance and harmony is called the holistic center (see Figure 2). The state of being holistically centered is when all three are dynamically in-sync, healthy, and nurturing to each other.

15

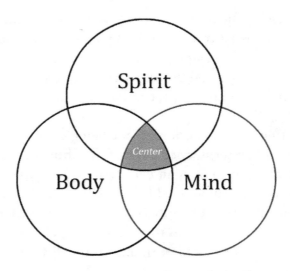

Figure 2: Holistic Center of Body, Mind, and Spirit

Being holistically centered gives us the power to face life's uncertainties with a sense of peacefulness and calm, without worry or fear. You've heard the term, being "off-center." Well, most of us live that way, but as we'll see in coming chapters, it's possible to achieve balance and live from that holistic center of your body, mind, and spirit anytime you choose—even when living with a debilitating illness like Lupus.

So, to live a beautiful life could be summed up this way:

Living a beautiful life means to live life to its fullest, finding a way to center oneself, holistically balanced in body, mind, and spirit, despite the trials and traumas of every day life.

An exciting prospect. Let's hold on to this thought as we explore what it means to live with Lupus—a complex, mysterious, and unpredictable illness.

PART II:
What Does It Mean
to Live with Lupus?

Chapter 3:
Systemic Lupus Erythematosus—An Overview

Living with Lupus, by its very unpredictable nature, challenges the body, mind, and spirit's ability to live holistically in harmony and balance. One doctor described Lupus as an autoimmune disease that attacks wherever blood flows the most. To me, that means it can strike anywhere at any time, regardless of how we live. And that's pretty much how it goes.

The official description of Systemic Lupus Erythematosus, also known as SLE or Lupus, is an autoimmune disease that can damage any part of the body—from skin and joints to major organs, like the heart, kidneys, lungs, and brain.[11] Like other autoimmune diseases—such as Rheumatoid Arthritis, Multiple Sclerosis, Myasthenia Gravis, Hashimoto's Thyroiditis, to name a few—the body's system for fighting disease goes haywire. The blood that normally produces antibodies to fight disease instead produces antibodies that attack the body's own healthy cells.

In Lupus, those misguided antibodies, called autoimmune antibodies, attach themselves to various areas of the body, causing pervasive inflammation that can lead to damage and very serious health problems.

Inflammation is a condition in which your body responds to injury, tissue or cell damage, or infection by becoming red, swollen, sore, and hot. Inflammation can occur openly as with the body's response to a cut or wound. It can also occur silently inside the body with vague symptoms, which results in feeling generally sick, exhausted, and feverish. It means that the immune system is working overtime, requiring lots of energy. Living in a constant state of inflammation is the cause of most autoimmune diseases, doctors say.[12]

The cause of the autoimmune inflammatory process is not totally clear to the medical community. After years of research, they know *what* is happening, but they still do not know *why*. And without the why, the disease remains a chronic condition that has no cure.

The Lupus Foundation of America reports that there are likely 1.5 million Americans and 5 million people around the world living with one of the four forms of Lupus:[13] 1) Cutaneous Lupus Erythematosus, which primarily affects the skin with lesions, rashes, scarring, and hair loss; 2) Drug-induced Lupus, which is caused by strong medications used to treat other diseases; 3) Neonatal Lupus, which affects infants whose mother's Lupus antibodies are transferred during gestation; and 4) Systemic Lupus Erythematosus, which affects various body systems and accounts for about 70 percent of all four types of Lupus.[14] This last type of Lupus, Systemic Lupus Erythematosus, is what I have been diagnosed with and what I'll focus on in this book. I will also shorten it to simply Lupus or SLE.

Lupus—Fact vs. Fiction
Many of us think we fully understand the disease and know all there is to know. While that might be true for some, there still may be some misconceptions out there. So, before continuing, it's important to understand and separate the facts from the fiction associated with Lupus.

First, the facts about Lupus:
1. Lupus is a chronic, never-ending autoimmune disease that is difficult to diagnose due to its many, seemingly unrelated symptoms.
2. Lupus presents itself differently in each person.
3. Lupus is an unpredictable disease of an on-again-off-again nature, meaning it flares up without warning and quiets itself just as suddenly.
4. Lupus flares can be caused by environmental triggers, such as exposure to UV rays, infection, overwork, injury, emotional or physical stress, pregnancy, and childbirth.
5. Some people with Lupus have a genetic predisposition to the disease.
6. Lupus is diagnosed based on an 11-criteria diagnostic evaluation developed by the American College of Rheumatology.
7. Women make up over 90 percent of the people living with Lupus.

8. Women of color (of African, Asian, or Hispanic descent) are at the highest risk of getting the disease.
9. No one knows what causes Lupus.
10. There is no cure for Lupus.
11. People with Lupus are living longer because of research and new therapies.
12. There has only been one new medication, Benlysta, approved for treating Lupus specifically within the last 50 years. Unfortunately, it was effective in only 35 percent of those who have taken it during clinical trials.[15] It has not been effective at all for African Americans with Lupus.[16]

Now the fiction:
1. "Lupus is contagious." Wrong—Lupus is NOT contagious. It is a non-communicable illness, which means it cannot be spread from one person to another.
2. "Lupus is like cancer or HIV/AIDS." Wrong—Lupus is not an infection, or a virus, or type of cancer. Lupus is an auto-immune disease where the body attacks itself, causing harm to major organs and body systems. Severe cases of Lupus are treated with the same chemotherapy drugs used to treat cancer; but Lupus itself is not cancer.
3. "Lupus only affects certain types of people." Wrong—Lupus can strike anyone at anytime, regardless of age, gender, or race.
4. "People with Lupus can't be that sick because they don't look sick." Wrong—Lupus can be a very disabling and potentially fatal disease that turns itself off and on. So, although people with Lupus can look good at a particular moment in time, they are suffering in ways that are not always visible.
5. "There are no effective treatments for Lupus." Wrong—Although there's no cure for the disease, Lupus can be treated effectively with medications and lifestyle changes, such as those outlined in this book.
6. "There's no need to educate people about Lupus." Wrong—Lupus continues to be a misunderstood disease, so it remains important to educate patients, caregivers, healthcare provid-

ers, and even doctors about the disease. Several non-profit organizations exist for the purpose of advocacy and awareness of the disease.[17] (See Resources on page 103 for a complete list.)

Diagnosis Code: 710.0

When I found out that I had Lupus, it wasn't the first time I'd heard of it. I knew of friends who had siblings, parents, and cousins with Lupus. Even my own paternal aunt suffered from the disease.

At different points over the years, I looked into whether or not Lupus could have been the cause of my many health problems. But because my symptoms included pulmonary embolism, chronic hives and angioedema, a torn sartorius muscle, pre-term labor, and avascular necrosis in both hips, I dismissed Lupus. No one else with Lupus had symptoms like mine. I was a *different* kind of sick. Or, so I thought.

Little did I know that Lupus presents itself differently in each and every person. No two cases are alike. That's why it's so difficult to diagnose.

None of my previous doctors in Washington, DC, Las Vegas, NV, or at UCLA Medical Center diagnosed it. Those who looked at my case as a whole suspected all kinds of other illnesses—from sickle cell anemia to sarcoidosis. Nothing panned out. All the tests were negative.

In the meantime, my conditions and episodes continued to pile up. My sickness résumé showed over 20 years of experience.

It wasn't until my husband and I moved from Las Vegas to Reno, NV that I finally got some answers.

I believe the answers finally came for two reasons: first, I had a fresh set of eyes looking at my case as a whole without judgment; and second, I had my medical records organized and summarized in one binder so that my new doctors could see for themselves the whole picture of my health history.

We moved to Reno in July 2012. Before we were completely settled in, I scheduled my first appointment with my new internist for August 21, 2012.

With my thick medical records notebook in tow, my husband and I met with the new internist. She was a very young and energetic woman who I felt comfortable with right away. I explained that I wanted to get established as a patient with her and that my case was a bit of a medical mystery, given all that I'd been through up to that point.

She honed in on the notebook, and she took her time going over everything in it. She said it was very helpful, as she "umm-hmmmed" her way through the pages.

Once she finished, she told us that she suspected an autoimmune disease, and she gave me a lab slip and sent us on our way.

Within two days of my blood draw at the lab, my new internist called to say that I tested positive for an autoimmune disease. At that time, she didn't say which one. My heart skipped a beat in that moment. Could this finally be it? The answers I've been waiting for?

She referred me to a rheumatologist, for whom I would have to wait over three months to see.

During that waiting period, I ordered a copy of my rheumatology blood tests. Abnormal results stood out for two tests—the ANA and the Anti-DNA ds.

These lab results were my first clue that the autoimmune disease could be Lupus. In my research to get more of an understanding of the disease, I came across the 11 criteria that doctors are instructed to use in diagnosing Lupus. According to the American College of Rheumatology, "a person is defined as having SLE if any four or more of the 11 criteria are present, serially or simultaneously, during any interval of observation."[18]

American College of Rheumatology
Criteria for Classification of Systemic Lupus Erythematosus[19]

1. Malar Rash: Fixed erythema, flat or raised, over the malar eminences, tending to spare the nasolabial folds. [A butterfly-shaped rash across bridge of nose and cheeks.]

2. Discoid Rash: Erythematous raised patches with adherent keratotic scaling and follicular plugging; atrophic scarring may occur in older lesions. [Raised red patches on your skin.]

3. Photosensitivity: Skin rash as a result of unusual reaction to sunlight, by patient history or physician observation.

4. Oral Ulcers: Oral or nasopharyngeal ulceration, usually painless, observed by physician. *[Ulcers and sores inside your mouth, including lips, gums, inside cheeks, tongue, throat, or nose.]*

5. Nonerosive Arthritis: Involving two or more peripheral joints, characterized by tenderness, swelling, or effusion. *[Arthritis, in the joints farthest away from the core of the body, that doesn't destroy the joints but causes tenderness and swelling from fluid build-up.]*

6. Pleuritis or Pericarditis: Pleuritis—a convincing history of pleuritic pain or rubbing heard by a physician or evidence of pleural effusion; OR Pericarditis—documented by electrocardiogram or rub or evidence of pericardial effusion. *[A build up of fluid or swelling in the lungs and lining of the lungs that causes pain and rubbing sounds (pleuritis); or a swelling of the lining around the heart (pericarditis).]*

7. Renal Disorder: Persistent proteinuria > 0.5 grams per day or > than 3+ if quantitation not performed; or Cellular casts—may be red cell, hemoglobin, granular, tubular, or mixed. *[Excessive protein in the urine, or abnormal microscopic cells in the urine.]*

8. Neurologic Disorder: Seizures—in the absence of offending drugs or known metabolic derangements; e.g., uremia, ketoacidosis, or electrolyte imbalance; or Psychosis—in the absence of offending drugs or known metabolic derangements, e.g., uremia, ketoacidosis, or electrolyte imbalance. *[Seizures and/or psychosis not caused by drugs or other physical or chemical imbalances.]*

9. Hematologic Disorder: Hemolytic Anemia—with reticulocytosis; or Leukopenia—< 4,000/mm3 on ≥ 2 occasions; or Lymphopenia—< 1,500/ mm3 on ≥ 2 occasions; or Thrombocytopenia—<100,000/ mm3 in the absence of offending drugs. *[Low red blood cell count (hemolytic anemia), low white blood cell count (leukopenia), low lymphocyte count, a type of white blood cell (lymphopenia), or low platelet count (thrombocytopenia) not caused by drugs.]*

10. Immunologic Disorder: Anti-DNA ds: antibody to native DNA in abnormal titer; Anti-Sm: presence of antibody to Sm nuclear antigen; Positive finding of antiphospholipid antibodies on: 1. an abnormal serum level of IgG or IgM anticardiolipin antibodies; 2. a positive test result for lupus anticoagulant using a standard method; or 3. a false-positive test result for at least 6 months confirmed by Treponema pallidum immobilization or fluorescent treponemal antibody absorption test. *[Blood tests reveal antibod-*

ies to double stranded DNA, to Smith nuclear antigen, or to cardiolipin.]

11. <u>Positive Antinuclear Antibody</u>: An abnormal titer of antinuclear antibody by immunofluorescence or an equivalent assay at any point in time and in the absence of drugs. *[A positive blood test for antinuclear antibodies (ANA) not caused by drugs known to induce it.]*

This list was shocking to me because I counted having a total of 7 of the 11 criteria—photosensitivity, oral ulcers, nonerosive arthritis, pleuritis, hematologic disorder, immunologic disorder, and positive test for antinuclear antibodies. And each of these happened at different times, spanning many years and each was treated by a different specialist and sometimes in different cities. No wonder no one made the connection.

Without my medical records notebook, my new doctor probably would not have been able to see the whole picture and suspect Lupus as she did. To learn about how to organize and assemble your own medical records notebook, see my article:

"How to Create Your Medical Records Notebook" at
www.liveabeautifullifewithlupus.com/medicalrecordsnotebook/

The more I continued reading and researching, the more I was able to associate my health history with the disease. My original assumption was that it all began with my pulmonary embolism in 2008. But, really, looking back, my body showed the beginnings of the disease as early as my teens. The bone pains, unexplained fevers, constant dry eyes, and strange infections all point to Lupus. Only with age, a difficult pregnancy, and blood clots in my lungs did the full picture begin to emerge.

The Lupus Foundation of America says it takes an average of four years and seeing three specialists before getting a Lupus diagnosis.[20] With so many varied symptoms and so much time between symptoms in my case, it took many more years than the average.

My first meeting with the rheumatologist went well. At the end of my appointment, she handed me a patient summary and a lab slip. In the section labeled "diagnosis codes," I saw an unfamiliar number—710.0. As my husband drove us home, I pulled out my smartphone and searched the Internet for its meaning. The 710.0 code represented "Systemic Lupus Erythematosus." With that, my Lupus diagnosis was finally official.

As twisted as it sounds, I was excited and thrilled to finally have a label for my failing health after all these years. It didn't take long, however, for my feelings of validation to turn to fear of what it would actually mean to live with Lupus.

—————————————————————————————————

For those of us living with Lupus, the damage the disease causes in the body as well as the mind affects the spirit. In the next few chapters, I will go over the specifics of how Lupus impacts each of the three dimensions of our lives.

Chapter 4:
How Lupus Affects the Body

The Lupus body is alarmingly delicate and sensitive. Many environmental, dietary, and emotional factors can trigger a worsening of symptoms that often leads to a fullblown flare of the disease. These flares, or episodes of worsening symptoms, manifest in the body as:

Pain: The pain from Lupus can be felt all over the body for many reasons. In the joints, from arthritis or avascular necrosis; in the muscles from myositis, tendonitis, myalgia, bursitis; in the chest from swelling of the linings of the lungs or heart; in the nerve fibers of hands, legs, and feet from peripheral neuropathy.[21]

Fever: Many of us with Lupus are more likely to experience elevated body temperatures or fevers that have no apparent source of origin.

Skin disfigurement and rashes: Lupus also creates devastating skin reactions that result in the commonly referred to "butterfly rash," with its raised lesions across the bridge of the nose and cheeks; large red and itchy autoimmune hives; temporary hair loss; discoid rash that leaves scarring in the scalp causing permanent hair follicle damage.

Oral Problems: Not so commonly talked about is how Lupus affects our oral health. Mouth sores on the tongue, inner cheeks, throat, and roof of mouth form for no reason, changing how we taste food and creating pain when we eat and drink certain ingredients.

Infections: Lupus patients suffer from recurrent infections and related complications because of our altered immune systems. Sometimes it's also due to immune-suppressing drugs that lower our resistance. Common infections in Lupus are yeast infections, colds and other upper respiratory infections, influenza, tuberculosis, and urinary tract and bladder infections.[22]

Swelling: With Lupus, it's no surprise to experience swelling in different parts of the body due to a build up of fluid in the joints of the hands, legs, and feet. Swelling can also present itself in the linings of the heart or lungs.

Fatigue: The exhaustion and fatigue that Lupus causes is one of its more debilitating effects on the body. It's difficult to explain to people how tired the disease makes you. The best descriptions I have are: "I feel like I've run out of gas, and there's nothing left, even in the reserve tank." Or, "I feel like I've been hit by an 18-wheeler—flat out and unable to get up."

Flares: The Lupus "flare" is an area of ongoing debate due to the lack of an agreed upon definition. Those in the Lupus patient community define a flare as a worsening of Lupus symptoms. But some in the medical community believe that definition to be too vague. They choose to apply a more scientific definition—one that can be measured in more quantifiable terms. For them, a flare is a worsening of symptoms that is confirmed with laboratory testing, radiological imaging, or a physician-conducted examination.[23]

Vital Organ Failure: As if the previously mentioned effects on the body weren't bad enough, Lupus can also lead to complete organ failure. This happens when those autoimmune antibodies launch a silent attack on the cells of the organs, slowly reducing function to the point where total failure occurs. Kidney failure, heart failure, reduced lung function, stroke, seizures, and reduced brain functionality, if left untracked and untreated, can lead to loss of life.

How Lupus Has Affected My Body

As of this writing, my doctors are referring to my current state of Lupus health as "stable"—meaning that the disease is still active, as evidenced by my continued abnormal autoimmune blood profiles and history, but stable because the medications and treatment I receive thankfully are managing to keep the Lupus autoimmune response from causing severe or life-threatening physical complications. We've achieved stability with:

1. A medication called Plaquenil, an anti-malarial drug that has done wonders to help with not only my fatigue and exhaustion, but also with reducing my episodes of autoimmune hives and angioedema (swelling of my lips and nose), pleurisy (inflamed lining of the sac surrounding my lungs), and related chest pain.

2. The blood thinner Coumadin to prevent any additional blood clotting issues that caused the pulmonary embolism in both lungs.

3. A weekly treatment regimen of physical therapy, massage, and acupuncture that focuses on managing the pain caused by headaches; arthritis; peripheral neuropathy in my legs, arms, and hands; avascular necrosis (bone death) in both femoral heads of my hips; and overall myositis and myalgia (muscle pain and inflammation).

4. Diligence in avoiding sick people and paying close attention to hygiene and food safety in order to avoid infection.

All of these have made a huge difference in how I am able to live with the effects of Lupus on my body. However, stability unfortunately doesn't mean that I'm free of symptoms. Even with medications and weekly treatment regimen, the pain is still a big issue, and I find my body dealing with symptoms that are more of a nuisance than life-altering. These include Raynaud's phenomenon, where my fingers turn blue for no reason; unexplained fevers; hair loss and scarring from lesions in my scalp; and painful, red mouth sores and ulcers.

Because of Lupus' effect on my body, I am a regular patient of 10 doctors: an internist, rheumatologist, neurologist, hematologist, cardiologist, pulmonologist, two orthopedists, a dermatologist, and otolaryngologist. They all monitor the part of my body that they specialize in, with my internist and rheumatologist overseeing it all. I liken it to a wheel with spokes—my internist and rheumatologist are in the hub and all my other doctors are the supporting spokes in the wheel that keeps me moving.

Chapter 5:
How Lupus Affects the Mind

The Lupus mind can suffer with the effects of the disease in both a psychological and neuropsychiatric, or brain chemical, sense. These affect the way we think, process, and perceive the world around us.

Experiencing constant pain, dealing with physical disfigurement, and the other bodily manifestations of Lupus can cause us to suffer emotionally and behaviorally with these conditions:

Depression: Sometimes, this is also thought of as an effect of changes in brain chemistry; but for the most part, depression in Lupus is due to the effects of treatments, medications, and living with a chronic disease. Some of us feel a prolonged deep sense of sadness and dejection.

Anxiety: This unsettled state of inner turmoil causes feelings of impending doom, dread, and fear. The unpredictable nature of Lupus leaves many patients feeling out of control, just waiting for the next flare or life-threatening episode to happen. This type of anxiety makes us generally fearful of the future.

Changes in Personality: Many of us with Lupus find that our reactions to everyday situations have changed. Our tempers are shorter, we feel lonely and isolated, and it's difficult to meet expectations of family, friends, and work associates. So, we withdraw and sometimes feel anger and resentment.

Inability to Handle Everyday Stress: The depression, anxiety, and/ or personality changes resulting from Lupus also cause the Lupus patient to lose the ability to handle the everyday stresses of life. By not handling stress, I mean reduced problem-solving and coping skills and a tendency toward denial and disengagement in order to avoid dealing with the stressors.[24] In addition, the fact that the Lupus is worsened physically and emotionally by the stress response itself only exacerbates the problem.

The Lupus mind is also affected by the biochemical abnormalities in the brain. These can impair neuropsychiatric function by causing decreased blood flow to the brain or by causing Lupus antibodies to cross the brain-blood barrier.[25] The neuropsychiatric effects of Lupus include:

Cognitive Dysfunction: Also known as "Lupus fog," cognitive dysfunction is the inability to think clearly. The periods of fuzziness come and go, and typically coincide with periods of higher disease activity.[26]

Memory Loss: When Lupus reduces blood flow to the brain, it can damage brain cells in memory storage areas. This causes memory loss and confusion that can get worse over time.

Psychosis: Reported in only about two percent of Lupus patients, psychosis is diagnosed when instability of brain chemistry causes delusion (false beliefs), paranoia, and/or hallucinations.[27]

How Lupus Has Affected My Mind

As a Lupus patient, I have experienced the neuropsychiatric effect of cognitive dysfunction from time to time; but, by far, the toll of the emotional and behavioral effects of depression and anxiety have been much greater.

Since taking Plaquenil, there has been a huge improvement in my charity of thought. It has made me less tired, which in turn made me less groggy, lifting the so-called Lupus fog. That's not to say that there aren't any times when I feel fuzzy. But for the most part, those times are few and far between as long as I'm getting the proper sleep and rest.

The treatment for depression and anxiety hasn't been so cut and dry. Over the years, pre- and post-Lupus diagnosis, I suffered with debilitating anxiety—fearful of everything and everyone, especially what my own body might do next. After the pulmonary embolism nearly took my life, my anxiety level was so high that I sought the help of a psychotherapist. After her evaluation and testing, she explained that I was suffering from generalized anxiety as well as depression due to my feelings of hopelessness surrounding my medical condition. This was prior to the Lupus diagnosis.

A few years later, just after receiving the Lupus diagnosis, the depression and anxiety returned as I was faced with what it meant to live with an unpredictable, incurable, and chronic disease. I began working with another psychotherapist who introduced me to tools to help

30

me cope, such as autogenic training and progressive neuromuscular relaxation. Both are forms of relaxation therapy that involve visualization and body awareness to facilitate a more controlled response to stress. (To learn more about these and other relaxation techniques, please see the Resources section on page 103.) We continue to work on emotional issues surrounding my health, mostly the impact of on-going, debilitating pain.

Chapter 6:
How Lupus Affects the Spirit

With the physical manifestations of Lupus on the body and the neuropsychiatric, emotional, and behavioral effects on the mind, the spirit of the Lupus patient often suffers as well. It's common for Lupus patients to feel disconnected from their beliefs in God, a higher power, or life force that gives meaning, hope, comfort, and inner peace to our lives. How can God let this happen? This is especially true when Lupus causes life-threatening episodes on one extreme and debilitating depression on the other.

The result is a spiritual emptiness that changes how we see ourselves in the world and how we define our purpose for living and being. Living in an atmosphere of spiritual powerlessness and hopelessness keeps us from realizing the fullness that life can offer. Lupus diminishes our spirit by:

1. Causing us to believe there is no hope.
2. Robbing us of inner peace.
3. Keeping us trapped, thinking we have no control.
4. Testing our faith because we don't know how to get better, and a return to whole health doesn't always happen.
5. Weakening our resolve.
6. Making us think of ourselves as a chronically ill person, instead of a whole person living with a chronic illness.
7. Disabling us from seeing the larger meaning of life and love, leaving us to limited social contact with friends and family support systems.
8. Lowering our expectations for possible positive outcomes in spite of the odds.

The good news is that by nurturing the Lupus spirit, we can treat it just as effectively and successfully as we treat the Lupus mind and body.

How Lupus Affected My Spirit
Lupus' impact on my spirit created in me a forced adaptation of how I found inner peace. Prior to the more serious worsening of

my health due to Lupus, I was able to connect to my spiritual self through techniques such as, deep breathing, yoga, and hiking in natural surroundings, such as deep forests, mountains, beaches, and lake shores. I loved taking pictures and breathing in the fresh air. These activities gave me a deep sense of calm and connectedness.

As my physical and emotional health deteriorated further, I found myself unable to reach the beautiful remote places in nature. The pain and other limitations of my body prevented that. I can no longer practice yoga due to the pain in my hips from the avascular necrosis. Even my deep breathing, centering meditative practice had to stop due to my constant pleuritic chest pain and the anxious thought that the pain could be another pulmonary embolism. Just about every one of my go-to spiritual practices had to be stopped or modified because of Lupus.

As a result, I began to question if my spirituality would ever be the same. The answer is that it won't. Facing that truth was difficult. But, as I began to consider other ways to connect spiritually, I began focusing on things that I could do, not what I could not do any longer. I increased my practice of prayer and, as suggested by my acupuncturist, I tried guided meditation that didn't rely so much on deep breathing.

Photography, another creative pursuit I would normally use to nurture my spirit became too difficult because of the arthritis pain and tremors in my hands and wrists. I thought of using a tripod, but having one more thing to carry was out of the question. In place of photography, I tried returning to calligraphy, which I enjoyed as a child; however, that didn't work for the same reasons. So, I decided to take up watercolor painting, something that I also enjoyed as a child, but didn't require as much precision. I found watercolors to be a way to literally flow with my limitations rather than fight them.

Throughout all the spiritual challenges of Lupus, I remained determined to find a way to kindle that joy and inner peace from my spiritual practice. Making these changes has done wonders for my spirit because I know that I can adapt no matter what I'm faced with.

PART III:
It's Possible to
Live A Beautiful Life with Lupus

Chapter 7:
The Power of Habits and Rituals

"We are what we repeatedly do. Excellence, then, is not an act, but a habit."
                                                                    ~Aristotle

Unfortunately, when the three dimensions of body, mind, and spirit are not in balance, due to physical disease, emotional or mental illness, or a disconnect within our spiritual lives, we are unable to find lasting happiness. It doesn't take much to throw off the balance, either. Even for the healthiest among us, daily stresses, sedentary lifestyles, and less than nutritious eating habits take a toll on us over time. Little by little, it wears away at us and our potential to live fully.

Healing the imbalance in the three dimensions takes more than addressing the individual dimension that seems to be suffering most, because each one affects the other two. With the advent of holistic medicine, the medical community has begun to collect a growing body of knowledge and evidence that supports the application of the total body-mind-spirit approach when treating diseases and maintaining wellness.[28] For example, treating the body for disease without addressing its impact on the mind will not be as effective. Add in the spiritual dimension of faith, prayer, meditation, or worship, and one can see how the healing process can be even more powerful.[29]

So with this scientific evidence showing the benefits of the body-mind-spirit approach to healing, we see that those of us living with a chronic disease, such as Lupus, the holistic healing approach must be applied in an ongoing way—not just in response to one illness event. We LIVE with illness events in one way or another every day, and relying only on prescription drugs to treat what ails the body and/or mind is not always the answer. Don't get me wrong; prescription drugs for Lupus have their place in keeping us functional and managing the risk of potentially deadly complications. God knows where I would be without my Plaquenil and Coumadin. But, to support our medicines, we have to learn specific rituals and habits to help us create an environment of holistic healing.

Before deciding to apply this holistic approach to my own Lupus body, mind, and spirit, I was living in what I call the "Lupus disconnect," where I reactively responded to my health needs based on which area was screaming the loudest. Going from reacting to the pain and physical issues of my body, to dealing with the mental stress and anxiety caused by the ups and downs of living with an unpredictable disease, to dismissing and ignoring my spiritual needs, I spent my life in the empty space somewhere between the three, as separate parts of myself.

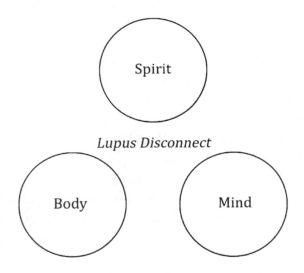

Figure 3: Lupus Disconnect of Body, Mind, and Spirit

Once I applied a more integrated approach to my health and healing, I found myself no longer reacting so much. Instead, I started taking a more proactive stance to managing the uncertainties of my life with Lupus. By proactive, I mean that I took specific steps to soothe my Lupus body, strengthen my Lupus mind, and nurture my Lupus spirit.

I created rituals and habits that naturally transitioned me from a state of "Lupus disconnect" to a unified body, mind, and spirit more capable of not only managing the Lupus, but also living a beautiful life with it.

These habits and rituals helped me to see Lupus for what it is—a manageable disease that I have some degree of power over. With the right medications and a commitment to the holistic healing of my body, mind, and spirit, I can and *will* live a beautiful life with Lupus.

What Are Habits and Rituals?

Habits and rituals basically describe the deliberate acts or series of acts that a person does in a repeated way.[30] [31] While rituals tend to be more ceremonial in nature (based on traditions, customs, and belief systems), habits are repeated acts that become second-nature behaviors.

For my life, rituals are the acts that allow me to honor and revere my three dimensions. Taking a soothing aromatherapy bath with candles and soft music is one of my rituals for soothing my Lupus body. Enjoying my sacred space with meditation and prayer is a ritual I choose to nurture my Lupus spirit.

On the other hand, habits are the acts I've come to do on a more unconscious level for a particular reason. One of my many habits for soothing my Lupus body is eating what's now being called a "clean diet" of fresh, preservative-free foods, and adding foods that are known to decrease inflammation, such as olive oil, salmon and leafy green vegetables.[32] To strengthen my Lupus mind, as one example, I make a habit of managing my expectations of myself and of the people in my life.

By adding these habits and rituals consistently, I began paying more attention to how I was living with Lupus. I have found beauty from taking the time for myself, setting boundaries, and recognizing my special place in this world. I also discovered that habits and rituals for each dimension actually support and enhance the others as well. This new awareness has had a tremendous effect on how I feel in all areas of my life—holistically.

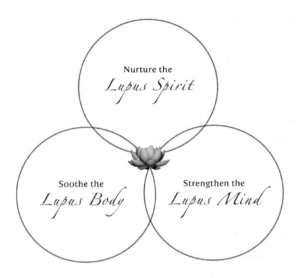

Figure 4: Living Holistically with Lupus—Body, Mind, and Spirit

Habits and Rituals that Unify
the Lupus Body, Mind, and Spirit— A Framework

To achieve this ongoing holistic healing, I had to develop a systematic approach to the whole idea of certain habits and rituals. I began documenting what I needed to do and understand about my body, mind, and spirit. From there, I developed the following framework of Lupus-targeted habits and rituals to soothe the Lupus body, strengthen the Lupus mind, and nurture the Lupus spirit—each dimension of my being contributing and elevating the other.

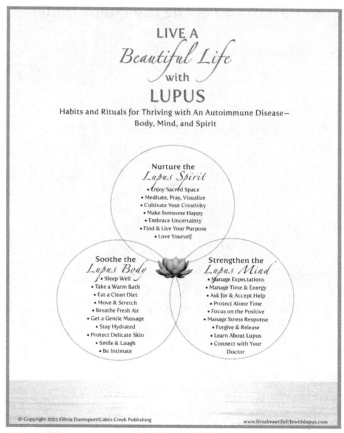

Figure 5: *Live a Beautiful Life with Lupus* Framework
For a free printable pdf of this *Live a Beautiful Life with Lupus* framework, please visit: *www.liveabeautifullifewithlupus.com/framework/*

The remainder of the book will examine each habit and ritual in depth to help you understand the importance and benefits of each and give you ideas and resources for making them a regular part of your life with Lupus.

Chapter 8:
Habits and Rituals to Soothe the Lupus Body

"Our body is a machine for living."

~Leo Tolstoy

The goal of practicing the habits and rituals to soothe the Lupus body (see Figure 6) is to increase your body's ability to operate more efficiently by what you subject it to internally and externally.

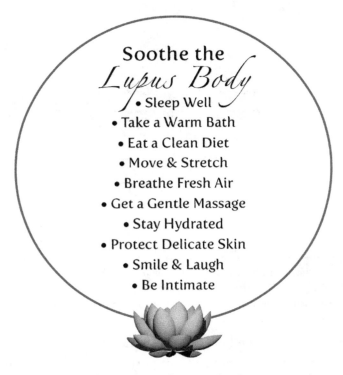

Figure 6: Habits and Rituals to Soothe the Lupus Body

Everything we do affects how our bodies respond to Lupus, so our actions should always be in line with minimizing pain, Lupus flares, and other physical manifestations of the disease.

Sleep Well

"Sleep is that golden chain that ties health and our bodies together."

~Thomas Dekker

Consistent, restful, and restorative sleep? What's that? The struggle to get the right amount of quality sleep—not too much and not too little—is still often daunting for me. Before Plaquenil did its job in helping with my exhaustion, I found myself sleeping like a cat, with long 12 or more hour stretches of sleep and intermittent napping. That was definitely too much sleep because I was groggy, cranky, and frankly not all there. My life was driven by that awful empty, no-energy feeling with nothing even in the "reserve tank." All I could do was sleep, and even sleep wasn't enough to relieve the fatigue.

Once my medication kicked in, though, I found myself having more energy; however, because the sleep hours were replaced with more activity, the arthritic, muscular, and neuropathic pain then became the deciding factor in my sleep pattern. My painful nights led to insomnia, limiting my sleep hours per night.

I'm not alone in my experiences with sleep. From not enough sleep to too much sleep to poor quality sleep—these are all common problems for us with Lupus. The Lupus Foundation of America cites several surveys showing that about 50 to 60 percent of Lupus patients report having sleep difficulties, which is consistent with surveys of other painful, chronic conditions.[33]

Our sleep problems aren't just an inconvenience. They actually have consequences of their own because of the role sleep plays in regulating our immune systems, which are already taxed and out of control. Too little sleep, researchers say, can increase inflammation, negatively affect the central nervous system, and increase sensitivity to pain.[34] Too much sleep throws off our sleep cycles and patterns causing us to sleep too much one night, and not enough the next.

According to the National Sleep Foundation, the recommended number of hours of sleep per night varies by age. Children need more because their bodies need the energy to grow. Adults between the ages of 18 and 65 should get between 7 and 9 hours of sleep per night in order to function well and have a productive and alert day. Over age 65, the recommendation goes down a bit to between 7 to 8 hours per night.[35] Most people, they acknowledge, can do well with a little more or a little less, as long as "you pay attention to your own individual needs by assessing how you feel on different amounts of sleep."[36]

For your best chance at understanding how much sleep you need in order to develop the habit of sleeping well—that is, getting consistent, restful, and restorative sleep—here are a few suggestions I compiled from the National Sleep Foundation and the Lupus Foundation of America:

- Establish a regular sleep schedule, even on the weekends.
- Eliminate distractions in your bedroom, like the television or the computer.
- Make sure your bed isn't contributing to your sleep problems. Be sure your bed linens are clean and your mattress supports your body's natural spinal alignment.
- If you are able, try to get regular exercise, but don't exercise in the evening too close to your bedtime. It may energize you and raise your core body temperature too much and interfere with your sleep pattern. (More about exercise in the "*Move and Stretch*" habit.)
- Turn off all electronics, including your smartphone, and lights before going to sleep.
- Don't eat heavy meals or drink alcohol within two to three hours of bedtime.
- Limit your daytime naps to no more than 30 to 60 minutes. Try not to nap after 5:00 pm.
- Limit the number of drinks and foods containing caffeine and other stimulants throughout the day, and do not consume them within two to three hours before bedtime.
- If pain at bedtime is an issue, consider sleeping with a microwavable body wrap, such as a Bed Buddy (found at Amazon.com). This has been a lifesaver for me on the many nights I lie down with pleuritic chest pain or arthritic joint pain.
- Get the correct pillow(s) to keep your spine aligned and to avoid putting strain or pressure anywhere on your body.

Take a Warm Bath

"I'm sure there are things that can't be cured by a good bath, but I can't think of one."

~Sylvia Plath

Ahhh, just the thought of sitting down in a warm bath soothes me. Notice I said *warm* bath—not hot bath. I make the distinction because I've found that if my bath water is too hot, it actually makes my condition worse.

Before Lupus, I loved hot baths, the hotter the better, especially after a good workout to soothe my aching muscles. Now, having lived with Lupus for a while, along with its neuropathic pain, autoimmune hives, and arthritic joints, I find hot baths to be painful. My body feels like it's on fire as my temperature rises.

As I looked into the possible reasons for hot baths becoming problematic, I discovered that heat sensitivity and intolerance are common in Lupus patients as well as others with autoimmune diseases. Heat worsens the inflammatory state of the Lupus body by increasing blood flow to areas that are already hot internally. While that might work to aid others who suffer muscle strain or injury, it's not the case with our bodies. It could be caused by the condition itself or the medications we take. Either way, hot baths aren't recommended, especially if you are experiencing a flare up of your symptoms.

So, after fearing that I would have to eliminate my bath rituals altogether, I tried lowering the temperature of the water. I've learned to get the benefits of a soothing bath with warm water—not much higher than my body temperature. Along with the correct water temperature, I sometimes add Epsom salts to help increase circulation (without the heat), relax my muscles, and ease joint pain. I forego the Epsom salts if my skin rashes are flaring up, though.

As opposed to taking a hot bath, a warm bath:
- Relaxes your body without activating the immune response of inflammation.
- Is closer to body temperature, making it more soothing to the Lupus body.
- Helps you sleep better than a hot bath if taken at night.

43

- Avoids raising body temperature too high, which can elevate your heart rate and cause stress on the cardiovascular system.[37] This is particularly problematic if Lupus has affected your heart function.
- Provides a more relaxing experience because warm water avoids revving up your nervous system the way a hot bath does.

To make the bath ritual even more soothing to the Lupus body, here are a few ways to enhance the experience:

- Add a few drops of essential oil to the water as it's filling the tub to create an aromatherapy atmosphere. Lavender or a citrus blend is relaxing. Be careful, though, not to slip in the tub with the presence of oils.
- Surround the bathroom and tub with tea light candles and soak in the tub by candlelight.
- Bring in 15 to 20 minutes of soft music. Create a bath time playlist on your smartphone, and start it just before stepping into your bath. By the time it's over, you should be sufficiently soothed.

Eat a Clean Diet

"Let food be thy medicine and medicine be thy food."

~Hippocrates

Like sleep, our choice of diet has a profound effect on the Lupus body. I know this first hand, having tried many diets to help deal with my brand of ongoing pain and inflammation. From vegan to Paleo to grain-free to gluten-free, I've experimented quite a bit. My goal with each diet trial was simply to feel better and manage the effect of my medications.

My conclusion, after all the trial and error? I feel best when I eat a clean, balanced diet, excluding foods that I know are problematic for me. Eating clean means eating, as much as possible, foods that are fresh, unprocessed or minimally processed. One rule of thumb for me is if it comes in a bag or a box, it's most likely processed, and I try my best to avoid it.

I do eat fresh fruits and vegetables, lean grass-fed meats (or as close to that as possible), fresh, wild-caught fish, and limited whole grains. Because beans and wheat/gluten-based breads and cereals are problematic for me, I exclude them. It's really been a process of elimination over the years while paying very close attention how I feel after eating certain foods. Keeping a food diary, although a huge pain, can be really helpful with this. (The *Lupus Diary*, described in Chapter 11, has a "Meals" section for this purpose.)

Mindless eating is no longer an option once you're diagnosed with Lupus. More important than taste or convenience, our choices of what to eat must be mindful of the goals of:

- Reducing inflammation and pain.
- Maintaining a healthy body weight.
- Avoiding deficiencies of nutrients, especially vitamin B-12 and vitamin D.
- Reducing the risk of heart-related complications of Lupus.
- Strengthening bones and muscles.
- Managing medication side effects.

With these issues in mind, I researched the recommendations of the Lupus medical and nutritional communities, and I compiled a list of what those of us with Lupus should eat, what we should not eat, and what we should test our Lupus body's response to.

Foods to Eat Abundantly

- Colorful fresh fruits and vegetables, both raw and cooked.
- Fresh, wild caught fish high in Omega-3 fatty acids.
- Lean, unprocessed, grass-fed meats, mostly poultry, lean pork, lean red meat.
- A variety of whole grains and beans, minimizing wheat and gluten.
- Healthy fats, such as seeds, nuts, and avocados.

Foods to Avoid Altogether[38]

- Alfalfa sprouts, which contain an amino acid that increases inflammation.
- Garlic, which contains compounds that increase immune system activity.

- Melatonin supplements, a sleep aid that stimulates the immune system.
- Echinacea, an herb that is used to boost the immune system, the opposite of what we need.
- Caffeine, which can overstimulate and affect the heart and central nervous system, which may already be affected by Lupus.
- Processed foods, such as frozen meals, which often contain both refined sugars, high sodium levels, and artificial ingredients and additives, which can worsen inflammation.
- Alcohol, which can interfere with your medication and cause the same inflammatory response as sugar.

Foods to Test How Your Lupus Body Responds
- Wheat and gluten-based foods. Try eliminating these breads, cereals, and other foods, such as soy sauce (which contains gluten) for one week to see if there's any decrease in pain and inflammation. These foods are known to cause inflammation in some of us living with Lupus and other autoimmune diseases. There are plenty of gluten-free and wheat-free substitutions available in grocery stores and online.
- Dairy products and cheeses. As with wheat and gluten-based foods, dairy products are also known to increase inflammation in some of us. So, try to eliminate these from your diet for one week to see if you feel any better. If you can't live without the taste, there are substitutions made with rice or coconut as the base, such as yogurts, cheeses, ice cream, and whipped cream. But be careful to read the label to make sure there is no "casein" in the ingredient list. Casein is a dairy product derivative used in dairy substitutes. Unfortunately, it can have the same detrimental effect as any pure dairy product.
- Salt and foods high in sodium. Lower your sodium content for a week to see if there is any improvement in joint swelling and mobility. Too much salt can cause you to retain fluid in your arthritic joints. Follow the guidelines for reducing sodium published by the American Heart Association.

Once you know which foods work for you and which foods cause more problems for you, you can tailor your clean diet accordingly. You'll begin to see food as an opportunity to nourish your body, not just satisfy empty cravings and hunger pangs.

Before making any changes in your diet, please discuss your plans with your doctors—your rheumatologist and your internist at the very least. They may have insights and precautions for you as you proceed. Your doctors may also refer you to a certified dietician or nutritionist who has even more expertise regarding how foods affect you and your particular case of Lupus.

Move and Stretch
"Movement is a medicine for creating change in a person's physical, emotional, and mental states."

~Carol Welch

Exercise for Lupus patients is one of those classic Catch 22 situations. We know that exercise is especially good for us for so many reasons, but we are often in too much pain or feel too tired to exercise. It's enough to drive you crazy or make you just give up—but don't do that.

I've discovered that it all has to do with our expectations of ourselves based on our history with exercise. What comes to your mind when you think about exercising? If you're like me, a formerly athletic person, you probably expect your body to do what it was once capable of. Initially, that drove my choice of exercises and workout times after learning I had Lupus. I often did too much and caused myself injury and pain, not understanding the effect it was having on me. Once I accepted my new Lupus body, without judging it, I realized that I needed help. I asked my doctor for a prescription for physical therapy so that I could learn how to exercise properly without hurting myself. My doctor sent me to a physical therapist who specializes treating the effects of autoimmune disease on the musculoskeletal system. My physical therapist tested the range of motion in my joints, suggesting further orthopedic testing based on my specific areas of pain, and generally encouraged me to move. She said it's the "moving" that matters and not to think of it as exercise.

That idea changed my whole mindset. And it gave me mental and emotional strength to adapt my movements even while using my cane or wheelchair as Lupus continued taking its toll on my body.

My physical therapist also explained that stretching and moving go hand in hand. Ever look at a cat when she wakes up from her naps? Well, our 12-year old cat always stretches just about every part of her body upon arising from her nap and before proceeding with her cat activities. She does the yoga cat pose, arching her back upward; then she stretches her front limbs with her butt in the air; from there, she stretches her facial muscles with a yawn; and finally, before scooting off, she stretches her back legs, one at a time. Same routine every time, multiple times a day. Her cat instincts know that stretching keeps her limber and agile, even as she ages.

There's a lesson in this for us humans with Lupus. Including stretching in our movement habit will only enhance the benefits of moving. You can choose to take on a full body stretching program, such as yoga, Pilates, or Tai Chi; or, if you're like me and that's just too much, you can start with focusing only on the major muscle groups—your back, neck, legs, chest, hips, shoulders, arms, and abdomen.

Without adding the habit of moving and stretching regularly, I know for sure that my Lupus body would be worse off. For those of us with Lupus, the benefits of this habit include helping us to:

- Fight Lupus fatigue.
- Strengthen the ability of our muscles to stabilize our swollen joints.
- Ease overall inflammation.
- Lift our mood.
- Improve flexibility.
- Extend the range of motion of major joints.
- Get out of bed with less pain.
- Decrease our chance of further injury.

Like all recommendations in this book, determine what works best for you by working with your doctor or other health practitioner. Here are a few suggestions for being successful in your moving and stretching[39] habit:

- See a physical therapist, preferably one who specializes in autoimmune diseases. S/he will help you develop a plan of moving tailored to your body's special needs. This will minimize the chance of injuring yourself.
- If you cannot go to a physical therapist, choose exercises that are soothing to your body. Pilates, yoga, and hydrotherapeutic (warm pool) exercises will do wonders to help you realize the benefits of moving.
- Be consistent once you get started on your habit of moving and stretching.
- Know when to stop—don't overdo it because you feel good.
- Know when not to exercise. If you have hot, swollen joints, rashes, or other signs of inflammation, it's best to hold off on the workout. On those days, exercise may wind up hurting more than helping you.
- Respect and accept your physical limitations. Build up gradually, if at all. Remember, the goal is to move, not train for a lofty goal right away. Who knows, with time, you may be able to run that 5K; but for now, it's baby steps, especially if you're not used to exercising or you live in constant physical pain, as I do.
- Avoid high impact, jarring exercises that compromise the joints or potentially tear fragile muscles.[40]
- Avoid bouncing as you stretch.
- Don't stretch cold muscles. Warm up with a shower, a slow walk, a warm pool, or any activity that warms the muscles that you plan to stretch.
- Don't push through pain. Ease up if anything begins to hurt.
- Breathe as you move and stretch. No holding your breath—you need to oxygenate your muscles as you move.

Breathe Fresh Air

"Fresh air impoverishes the doctor."

~Danish Proverb

Are you getting enough fresh outdoor air? For most of us with Lupus, whether we're working regularly or not, the answer is likely no. We're probably spending our days cooped up in our closed homes, cars, or offices, getting air only as we transition from one place to another. We might do better if the weather is warm and sunny, but that's not enough to reap the benefits of consistent amounts of fresh air. It's preferable to get fresh air in green spaces, where there are plenty of trees, where the air is clean as opposed to a city environment where the air is more likely to be polluted. If you can't get out of the city, find a nice park within city limits. To find out how clean or polluted the air is where you are, use AirNow at www.airnow.gov. AirNow issues daily air quality index (AQI) data and forecasts for over 400 U.S. cities and warnings about when the AQI could be bad for your health.

Fresh air benefits us by:[41]

- Improving the cleansing action of our lungs by bringing more oxygen to the cells, with each inhalation. With each exhalation, airborne toxins are released from your body.
- Improving your sense of well-being and ability to relax by providing oxygen to the serotonin stores in your body. Serotonin is a neurotransmitter that is responsible for regulating our moods, our appetite, ability to sleep, memory, etc.[42]
- Improving your heart rate and blood pressure. With more oxygen, your body doesn't have to work as hard. It's best to be in green spaces, amongst the trees, to receive this benefit; outdoor air that is polluted has the opposite effect.
- Sharpening the mind by supplying the brain with needed oxygen and giving our brains a break from our mentally draining lives.
- Helping with food digestion, which is important for us who take medicines that often interfere with this bodily function. The oxygen provides our bodies with oxygenated blood flow to our digestive tract, and that encourages efficient intestinal action.[43]

Here are a few ideas to help you get more fresh air:

- Take your "*Move and Stretch*" habit outside, in your back-yard, the park, a high school track—before or after school hours, of course.
- Get dirty in your garden, planting flowers or herbs and vegetables to support your "*Eat a Clean Diet*" habit.
- If it's safe to do so, sleep with your window open to allow more fresh air into your home at night.
- Sit on your front porch or stoop.
- Go to a non-smoking outdoor café that serves healthy, fresh food.
- Drive to your nearest lake shore or beach.

Get a Massage

"Your body is precious. It is your vehicle for awakening. Treat it with care."
~Buddha

For the Lupus body, massage can be a very welcome and soothing approach to pain relief. When expert hands release knotty muscles surrounding arthritic joints, they also release endorphins, those hormones known for relieving pain. Massage can also reduce inflammation and decrease soreness for those of us who suffer from more specific conditions, like myositis, fibromyalgia, or arthritis.

There's another side to the massage story that is important to understand when considering it for Lupus. First, if your Lupus manifests with any form of peripheral neuropathy, be careful before proceeding. Peripheral neuropathy is the result of damage to the nerves farthest away from the center of your body, mainly your arms, hands, legs, and feet. In my case, going for so many years with no Lupus diagnosis left my nerves exposed to the damaging effects of chronic, untamed inflammation. As a result, I sometimes experience peripheral neuropathy in all four areas at once.

Naturally, the nerve pain and numbness of peripheral neuropathy results in a different reaction to massage and touch in general. Either it's too painful to tolerate or the numbness creates a strange, not-so-pleasurable sensation.

51

This doesn't mean that massage is out of the question if you have peripheral neuropathy. It just means that you need to work with a massage therapist who has experience with this and other issues related to autoimmune disease.

Keep these tips in mind when considering using massage to soothe the Lupus body:

- Be aware of any signs of impending flares, rashes, lesions, or fever. If any of these issues are happening, postpone your massage until your body settles down and becomes stable again.
- Ask for gentle massage and avoid the deep tissue massage, which can aggravate your Lupus body. If you believe you would benefit from a deeper massage for certain areas, ask your massage therapist to go slow.
- Inform the massage therapist of your medications, especially if you're taking corticosteroids.
- Before each massage, give your massage therapist a run down of what's going on with your body and what you want to get out of the session.
- Let your massage therapist know if you experience any pain or discomfort during the session.
- Always, always, always work with a licensed and registered massage therapist, preferably one who specializes in working with clients who have an autoimmune disease. Ask around at your physical therapist's or doctor's office, where they will likely know of massage therapists who are more medically oriented. You can also search the website of the American Massage Therapy Association, using their locator service. Also check with your state's massage licensing organization to determine if the massage therapist you're considering is licensed by your state.
- Drink extra water after your massage. The rule of thumb for this purpose is to divide your body weight by two, and drink that number of ounces of water within 24 hours after your massage. For example, I weigh 130 pounds, which divided by two equals 65. I should drink 65 ounces of water within 24 hours after getting my massage.

- Avoid drinking caffeine and alcohol (which you should be avoiding anyway) for 48 hours after your massage; they are dehydrating and counteracting to the hydrating and cleansing effects of water.
- Take a warm bath with Epsom salt to aid in relieving possible soreness and release muscle tension. Add one to two cups of Epsom salt in a full tub of warm (not hot) water.
- Check with your health insurance to find out if you're covered for massage therapy. Many insurers are now including full or partial coverage of what they call alternative therapy sessions in their annual list of benefits.

Stay Hydrated

Drinking water for me often feels like a chore. It's not because I don't like the tastelessness of it; it has more to do with remembering to drink it. This remains true even with knowing how important it is. And, I'm not alone. An April 2013 study published by the U.S. Centers for Disease Control and Prevention shows that nearly half of us aren't drinking enough water. Forty-three percent of Americans drink fewer than four cups per day. That's far short of the recommended average amount of eight cups per day. The exact amount that's best for us, of course, is dependent on our physical build, activity level, and health circumstances.[44]

Either way, hydration is extremely important. For the Lupus body, remaining hydrated—with water and high-water content foods—is even more crucial. It's the number one, safest way to support our body's detoxification functions—breathing through our lungs; perspiring through our skin; urinating through our kidneys; and defecating through our intestines.

Without water and hydration, our bodies not only have to work harder to be rid of the by-products of our medications and other toxins and impurities that we're exposed to, it also suffers the damage of prolonged exposure to them. This only exacerbates the inflammatory response that is at the core of our disease.

Sometimes, dehydration can be the direct cause of your headache, dry mouth, dark urine, muscle cramps, or fatigue. It's so easy to blame Lupus for many of our ailments, but before you do, try drinking more water. I have to give my Hubby credit for helping me realize this. Every time I'd complain of a headache, his response was, "Are you drinking enough water today?" More often than not, I wasn't. And, when I did, sometimes the headache actually went away. (Not every time because there are headaches, and then there are head ACHES.)

So, to help your Lupus body stay hydrated, here are a few guidelines and tips:[45]

- Every day, drink 8 cups of water as a baseline; then add 1 to 3 cups of water for every hour of physical activity.[46] (Just for the record, 1 cup equals 8 ounces of water.)
- Do not wait until you're thirsty to drink. By then, you're likely dehydrated already.
- Drink before, during, and after your *"Move and Stretch"* habit.
- Carry a travel water bottle with you whenever possible.
- Infuse your water with fruit, if taste is an issue for you. Lemons in particular have helpful astringent and antioxidant properties that boost water's elimination benefits.
- Drink more water during a flare, especially if you're feverish or have an infection.
- Eat high water content foods as a regular part of your diet. Vegetables, such as cucumbers, spinach, lettuce, celery, and tomatoes; and fruits, like grapes, grapefruit, pineapples, cantaloupe, watermelon, and pears—all have 90 percent or more water content.[47]

Protect Delicate Skin

Lupus attacks our skin in many ways. Of the 11 criteria for diagnosing Lupus by the American College of Rheumatology (see pages 22-24), four involve skin conditions—malar (butterfly) rash across the bridge of the nose and cheeks, discoid rash, photosensitivity, and oral and nasal ulcers. In addition to these, many of us with Lupus also experience hair loss or alopecia, chronic autoimmune hives, Raynaud's phenomenon, purpura, cutaneous vasculitis, etc.

Strangely enough, many of the skin manifestations of Lupus are either caused or aggravated by exposure to the sun—specifically its UV rays. UV rays not only produce rashes, they also could cause an increase in the production of the autoimmune antibodies responsible for Lupus.[48]

So protecting our skin must become a daily habit. Here's how:

- *Sunscreen.* Not just any sunscreen. The most effective sunscreens are those with high, broad-spectrum sun protection factors or SPFs. Apply sunscreen on your face and anywhere else on your body that's exposed to the sun. My doctor recommended a broad-spectrum sunscreen with at least an SPF of 35. The consistent application of sunscreen has made a huge difference for my hands and face especially. These areas are exposed to very bright sunshine when I drive during the day, causing painful rashes and inflammation.

- *Sun-protective clothing.* In addition to sunscreen, wearing clothing made from fabric with built-in sun protection, especially covering the chest and arms, will provide a convenient and less messy option. You can even add sun protection to clothing you already own by adding to your laundry wash cycle a UV protectant, which does not damage your clothing.

- *Vitamin C moisturizer.* Non-irritating moisturizers with vitamin C also protect the skin by overcoming dryness, neutralizing free radicals, and reducing redness and inflammation. Don't start out using too much, though, because it can cause irritation in some of us who are especially sensitive to it.

- *Wear a hat.* So simple and easy to do. It gives extra protection to your face, which is the area of your body that is most exposed to the sun's harmful rays.

- *Use an umbrella.* If you have to be out and about in the sun for a prolonged period, shield yourself with an umbrella. Yes, it may seem a little weird to some, but your sensitive Lupus skin is more important than what others think.

- *Tint your car windows.* Living out in the western U.S., I've come to appreciate darkened car windows that provide additional glare reduction and sun protection for my skin. If only I could tint my windshield along with the rest of my windows.

Smile and Laugh

"Laughter is inner jogging."

~Norman Cousins

This habit might seem to be better suited under the next chapter, *Habits and Rituals for the Lupus Mind*, but I assure you that this is one for the body.

Have you ever heard of Norman Cousins? Well, he was a writer and editor for a now-defunct magazine called the Saturday Review back in the 1970s. He developed a rare, life-threatening autoimmune disease and was at the point where doctors had begun to expect the worst. While in the hospital, suffering from debilitating pain, Cousins began to notice how he felt better during and after visits with family and friends. He discovered that it was during those visits that he smiled and laughed deeply. The joy of it was one thing, but he realized there was a direct relationship between that deep belly laughter at the jokes of friends and family and how he felt physically. So inspired by this, Cousins wrote the book, Anatomy of An Illness, where he describes how he implemented "laughter therapy," in the form of comedic movies, to help him heal and recover from the disease.[49]

Although the use of humor in medicine goes back as far as the early 13th century, Cousins is credited with sparking real scientific research into the effect of laughter and humor on physical well-being. Some hospitals and medical treatment centers include laughter therapy as part of their physical therapy and exercise programs, believing that activating the muscles used in laughter will produce similar physical benefits.

For the Lupus body, laughter and humor therapy helps us to:
- Enhance our oxygen intake.
- Stimulate heart and lungs.
- Relax muscles throughout the body.
- Trigger the release of pain-killing endorphins, the hormonal response for pain relief.
- Ease digestion.
- Improve mental functions of clarity, memory, and alertness.
- Produce a sense of overall well-being.

Intuitively, I believe most of us know and understand this. Many people ask me why or how I can smile so much while living in so much pain. My usual answer is that I have to. It's the only way for me to live.

Be Intimate

"The need for love and intimacy is a fundamental human need, as primal as the need for food, water, and air."

~Dean Ornish

The disappearing physical closeness of a spouse or partner is all-too-often an unspoken area of suffering related to the Lupus body. The obvious issues of pain and fatigue aren't the only reasons for this. Other physical symptoms, such as rashes, lesions, oral ulcers, hair loss, infection, and medication side effects also contribute to our feeling less than desirable and unwanted on our end. For our spouse or partner, it could be that they're unsure of how or when or whether it's even safe to approach us for physical intimacy, given our many ongoing, chronic Lupus-related issues.

The natural, easy flow of sharing love physically becomes an awkward and frustrating void that we try not to think about. But, there are too many benefits of this area of our lives to just dismiss it.

First, let us consider exactly what intimacy is. Intimacy is more than sexual intercourse, although that can be a significant part of it. Intimacy is feeling an emotional and physical connection with a spouse or companion, where there's a shared sense of being loved, nurtured, safe, vulnerable, and content. Intimacy is where we fully share who we are without worry of judgment, and it often helps to define our place in the world.

Behaviors such as physical touch, eye-to-eye contact, smiles, compliments, unspoken communication, and sex reinforce the intimacy and help it to grow deeper over time.

Why is intimacy important to our physical well-being? Physical intimacy offers health benefits beyond the emotional aspects. From simple hugs and cuddling all the way to full on intercourse and orgasm, physical intimacy benefits us by:[50]

- Relieving pain with the release of endorphins.
- Improving sleep.
- Counting as part of the *"Move and Stretch"* habit.
- Helping us to maintain healthy blood pressure.
- Helping us to regulate the immune system.
- Relaxing muscles and releasing tension in the body.
- Helping with physical effects of stress and anxiety by stimulating oxytocin release while lowering our heart rate and cortisol levels.
- Reducing the risk of heart attack.

Because intimacy is such an important aspect of our adult lives, we must redefine, together with our spouses and partners, what intimacy means while living with Lupus. Here are a few steps to help bring back that wonderful aspect of your life together:

1. Start on common ground. Discuss how important that physical connection is to you both, what it means to you, and the aspects of the connection that are most pleasurable to you.

2. Touch and hug to maintain that physical connection. Even if it's awkward at first. Just do it.

3. Develop a shorthand communication, where you signal your partner when sex and intimacy are welcome and when it's best to wait. It spares you both from feeling shy about broaching the subject. My husband and I decided our signals would be in my selection of a certain nightgown for when I'm feeling up to it; and full-coverage pajamas for when I'm not.

4. When you are feeling up to physical intimacy, it helps to use pillows in strategic places to minimize the impact of intercourse. Under the hips and neck, if on your back or under your belly if you're on your side or stomach.

5. Plan for quality time together in the form of date night or date day. This way, you can plan your meds, your rest, and other considerations around your planned date time.

6. Take a soothing warm bath or shower together.

7. Try different positions to make intercourse less painful and more pleasurable.

8. If massage isn't too painful, include it during your times of intimacy.
9. Remain loving and positive, even on your worst days.

Track Your Lupus Body with the Lupus Diary

Use the *Lupus Diary* (see full description and link to your free copy in Chapter 11) to track what's happening with your Lupus body—your current symptoms, flare details, other physical episodes. Also track your successes and/or challenges with the habits and rituals to soothe the Lupus body listed in this chapter.

Chapter 9:
Habits and Rituals to Strengthen the Lupus Mind

"You have power over your mind – not outside events. Realize this, and you will find strength."

~Marcus Aurelius

Lupus drains not only our bodies, but also our minds. From the biochemical abnormalities that cause cognitive deficiencies, to recurring feelings of depression, anxiety, and stress, the effects of Lupus on our minds can be devastating and mentally depleting. Couple that with the responsibilities of every day life, and you have the recipe for feeling completely overwhelmed at the least; or worse, you experience relapse, flares, or a complete physical breakdown.

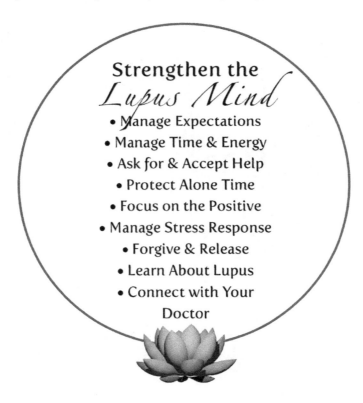

Figure 7: Habits and Rituals to Strengthen the Lupus Mind

The goal, once you become stable with the medications or treatments for your body, is to do no harm mentally. That is, keep the balance and do nothing to create a relapse of your symptoms. Lupus is unpredictable enough without our own actions contributing to it.

The objective of these habits and rituals to strengthen the Lupus mind is to help you manage your emotions and behaviors so that you minimize Lupus flares, brain fog, and other mental manifestations of the disease (see Figure 7).

Manage Expectations

Realizing that Lupus will have an effect on everything that I do for the rest of my life, I had to learn to manage my expectations of myself and others.

My feelings and standards about what I should achieve in a day, a month, a year, or in my lifetime for that matter, drastically changed.

Before Lupus, I was so accustomed to setting the bar exceptionally high for myself—in business, in physical training, in child rearing, in just about everything. I was literally Super Woman. A single Mom who worked full-time at my day job, I earned a master's degree part-time on the weekends, then served as an adjunct professor also on the weekends. I also found time to get a personal trainer certification, to date occasionally, to go to church regularly, and spend time with my son at dinner every night. Even as the symptoms and episodes of Lupus knocked me down a few pegs, I'd get back up, adjust, and continue living life, expecting to achieve, achieve, and achieve some more.

After a few life-threatening episodes, however, I was hit with a sudden dose of reality—the reality that my body would never be as it was before. Of course, I was devastated. On the flip side of that, however, I thought about how thankful and fortunate I was to be alive. That gratitude helped me change my expectations of myself. I began to see that life actually does go on without the need to out-do and outpace the world.

I began to look at why I put so much pressure on myself, and like most people my reasons included:

- Gaining the respect and approval of others.
- Thinking that achievements would lead to a happy life.
- Proving my doubters that they were wrong about me.
- Setting a good example for my son.

Once I discovered my reasons for setting the bar so high, I could "reset" my expectations of myself and move forward with a new mindset. It's not that I lowered my expectations; rather, I saw the flaws in what was motivating me to achieve them. Once I did that, it was no longer the priority to prove doubters wrong or even gain the respect of others. The priority became living a beautiful life with a chronic disease.

With this new priority in mind, I decided that I also had to change what others expected of me—my family, my friends, my employer. They were so accustomed to the old Olivia, the resilient one who always bounced back from adversity to get the job done no matter the cost.

Just as I had to look at what motivated my expectations of myself, I began to look at what motivated everyone else's expectations of me. I saw that their motivations fell into one of two camps: either they were selfish and self-serving for them or they were based on wanting what's best for me. Getting them to understand my illness and what it means for my life took time and effort. Based on my experience, here are a few tips to guide you in managing the expectations of yourself and others:

- *Challenge your expectations of yourself.* What's motivating them? Are they realistic? Are they even necessary given your challenges with Lupus?
- *Talk to those setting expectations of you.* Do they understand the disease and what it means to live with Lupus? Do they know your specific limitations?
- *Seek the counsel of a therapist or trusted family member or friend.* This will help you to gain strategies more specific to your life and situation and gain the confidence to put your needs first.
- *Express your feelings in a journal or diary.* (See the *Lupus Diary* in Chapter 11).

- Practice saying no in a kind way. Be prepared to do so when the expectations of others are not good for you and your health.
- Learn to live with a new set of limitations. Realize that you can meet your goals in a new way without giving up on them entirely in most cases.
- Take a break from those who have expectations of you. It's helpful to withdraw and get perspective about their motives.

Over time, those who fall into the camp of "wanting what's best for you" will adapt. All others will fall away, and that's okay.

Manage Time and Energy

For those of us with Lupus, time and energy are precious commodities, inextricably linked. The way you organize and plan your time has a deep effect on your energy levels; and your energy levels determine how you're able to spend your valuable time.

With this in mind, you have to spend a little time planning and managing both. It's important to remember that good time management must focus on results, not just the activities themselves.

So, what do you need to accomplish with your time and energy? What's most important for you to do? Will you have enough energy to do it? For example, as a single Mom, I often focused on the activity of cooking dinner, even when my energy levels were not up to it. If I had focused instead on the result of feeding my son and myself and spending quality time together at the end of the day, I would have realized that buying a prepared meal or a meal I'd prepared and frozen earlier would accomplish the same result. It certainly would have taken less of my energy.

Focusing on the results we need to achieve with our management of time and energy, we're better able to:
- Prioritize our responsibilities—what's important, instead of just being busy with familiar activities.
- Know when it's okay to stop if circumstances change.
- Better understand our limits and pace ourselves accordingly.
- Develop tools and systems for streamlining the process for getting those results. Tools and systems include:

- A central calendar, online or on the wall, to remind you of events, doctor appointments, when to take medications, run errands, etc.
- A magnetized list pad on your refrigerator to make note of when grocery items and toiletries run out.
- A pillbox to organize your daily medications and supplements.
- An organized and simplified home, especially closets, pantry, dressers to help you locate needed items without wasted time and energy searching.

The result of efficient time and energy management on the Lupus mind is that we:

- Deal more effectively with the neuropsychiatric effects of Lupus, better known as brain fog.
- Experience less stress because we're spending our time and energy wisely.
- Avoid the vicious cycle of going from Energizer Bunny to wet noodle—that is, working to the point of exhaustion on a good energy day only to be completely incapable of any task on the following day because we're too tired from the day before.

Ask for and Accept Help

Even with learning to manage our time and energy by understanding the desired results, we Lupus patients often find ourselves unable to accomplish all we need to do. Certain low-priority tasks fall off the radar. Or, when we're having a particularly difficult flare or unexpected illness episode, we're not even capable of meeting our top priorities in life.

It's during those times that we need to ask for and accept the support of family, friends, and others we trust.

For those of us who have been fiercely independent for most of our lives, asking for help goes against every fiber of our being. It makes us feel weak and vulnerable and beholden to others. It feels like we've lost control and are becoming a burden to those around us.

For me, I even held back asking my own husband for help, mainly because I didn't want to be a burden to him. By obstinately trying to do things on my own—instead of asking for his help and rejecting his offers to help—I often wound up hurting myself or facing regret for trying to do it all alone.

My mind changed when I talked with my friends about it. Knowing both my husband and me, these ladies all agreed that he would be delighted to help me, and that by shunning his offers, I was denying him an opportunity to show his love. Talk about shifting the focus from myself!

It's the same principle when you consider asking for and accepting help from others. When you don't ask or you shun offers, you are:

- Saying that their help isn't good enough for you.
- Denying them the opportunity to experience the happiness that comes from giving.
- Demonstrating that you are not trusting of them.
- Missing the opportunity of experiencing love and friendship on a whole new level as a vulnerable, imperfect human being.

The act of asking for and receiving support should also be practiced with your doctor or other health professional. Let them know when you're struggling. They may suggest that you seek support from a psychotherapist or community support group to connect with others with Lupus.

Help and support is often just a phone call away. Get beyond yourself and find the courage to simply ask. Then, graciously accept. Your Lupus mind will thank you.

Remember the saying, "It takes a village to raise a child?" Well, it also takes a village to live a beautiful life with Lupus.

Protect Your Alone Time

After having many episodes of severe illness and hospitalizations with Lupus, I discovered that the times I spent alone in recovery at home were especially nourishing to me. I paid attention to how I was feeling, and I kept a watchful eye on my body's healing. I was the priority during those times. But once I was able to get up and about again, that alone time fell off the radar because I had to get back to life—the never-ending routine of work, school, parenthood, church, etc.

During the most recent recovery, I decided to find a way to add my alone time to my busy life on a regular basis. I mean, why did I only get quality time alone with myself when Lupus knocked me down?

In my research about the importance of alone time, I found there are many mental health benefits that ring even truer for those of us with Lupus. Alone time gives you quiet time to:

- Get a better understanding of yourself.
- Replenish and rejuvenate your mind.
- Enjoy an atmosphere without pressure.
- Find solutions to ongoing problems.
- Slow down and relax.
- Explore possibilities for your future.
- Clear your mind of negative thoughts.
- Gain a fresh perspective.
- Simply do nothing (my favorite).
- Get away from the people who drain you emotionally.
- Take time away from conflicts.
- Sort out your feelings of anxiety, exhaustion, and depression.

Understanding that making alone time for yourself isn't always easy or comfortable, here are a few thoughts about how to make it a reality in your busy life:

- Make it a priority by adding it to your schedule. Start with just 15 minutes a week and work your way up to one hour, several times a week if possible.
- Combine alone time with another habit or ritual—such as a warm bath that soothes your Lupus body.
- Don't allow feelings of guilt to stop you. You deserve and need alone time.
- Become accountable to yourself.
- Keep track of your alone time with your *Lupus Diary* (see Chapter 11).
- Remember that it doesn't matter what you do, just make it a habit to get your "alone time" fix on a regular basis.

You have the right to recharge, replenish, and restore. Just as sleep replenishes the Lupus body, taking alone time replenishes the Lupus mind. It helps regain clarity and focus. It gives us calm in the storm taking place in our bodies as we try to manage life with a chronic disease.

Focus on the Positive

"Guard your mental house so that no negative thoughts find entrance."

~Unknown

I know this is one of those oversimplified, often-talked-about habits that sounds simple enough, but isn't simple for everyone.

How do you focus on the positive when Lupus is unpredictably wreaking havoc as it pleases? Positive thoughts are hard to come by sometimes, especially when you're fighting just to make it through a day or a given situation.

I'm happy to say that even with Lupus, it's possible to focus on the positive. In fact, I discovered it's even more crucial to do so, when you consider how negative thinking actually contributes to our illness. Haven't you noticed how you feel worse when you're dealing with negative emotions? For me, my pain levels explode when I'm angry or worried about something.

There's a reason for that. Specifically, negative thoughts cause more problems for systems already vulnerable to damage from Lupus:

- The cardiovascular system suffers from a surge in adrenaline production, which increases our heart rate and blood pressure.
- The respiratory system suffers from shallow breathing or breathlessness, affecting our intake of oxygen to our lungs and blood cells.
- The musculoskeletal system has to deal with our tense and strained muscles.

Until I learned to control my thoughts, I was at the mercy of them. And, I felt helpless to find a way to routinely focus on the positive in my life.

In order to take control so that I could focus on the positive, I had to understand and replace the negative. Only then, could I clean house, so to speak, and replace the negative thoughts with positive ones.

I've experienced the following three prevalent types of negative thinking because of Lupus—the inner critic, the worrier, and the all-or-nothing thinker.

Inner Critic. The inner critic thinks constant negative thoughts about herself caused by low self-esteem, lack of self-love, repeated self-rejection, and self blame when things go wrong in life. And, as we know, plenty can go wrong with Lupus. Because Lupus often prevented me from achieving the high goals and expectations I set, I began criticizing myself whenever I fell short. And, with time, the voice of the inner critic grew louder and louder. My therapist helped me to control these thoughts by encouraging me to catch and interrupt the self-deprecating thoughts. I made time to listen to my thoughts during alone time, and I began writing them down. It was startling to see on paper how poorly I thought of myself. My therapist encouraged me to replace the negative inner critic thoughts by telling myself how much I love and approve of myself—just as I am. No one is perfect, and we all make mistakes. It's not anyone's fault that I have Lupus. The same is true for you. If you recognize this inner critic negative thinking in yourself, I encourage you to work with a therapist or support group to help you stop putting yourself down.

Worrier. The worrier thinks negative thoughts caused by living in the world of what-ifs, and doing all she can to control and prevent the what-ifs from happening. This type of negative thinking is common with those of us with chronic, unpredictable diseases. We worry about when we'll have our next flare or major life-threatening episode. Like inner critic thinking, you can control worrier negative thinking by interrupting the thoughts and remembering how it is bad for your health—the health that you're so worried about. Worry prolongs anxiety in the mind and creates the fight or flight stress response in the body—both of which exacerbate the symptoms of Lupus. Replace the worrier negative thoughts about the future with thoughts of gratitude about the future. Be thankful for and envision stable health in the future. "What you see is what will be," as the saying goes. Positive visualization decreases the impulse to worry and the need to overreact to fear. (See the *"Meditate, Visualize, Pray"* ritual in Chapter 10.)

All-or-Nothing Thinker. With my high-achiever personality, I was guilty of perfectionism and the resulting all-or-nothing thinking long before my Lupus diagnosis. As I explained earlier, I lived a life of high expectations, even as a child. This way of thinking led me to create unrealistic expectations of myself. With my compromised health and ultimate Lupus diagnosis, I became less and less able to live up to those expectations. And, for a long time, I could only see my inability to reach my goals as a complete and total failure on my part. There was only success or failure—no in between. My mother calls it black-and-white thinking without acknowledging the gray areas of life. It's taken a lot of work to get out of this mindset to realize that my all-or-nothing thinking wasn't serving me as I managed my life with Lupus. Really, it didn't serve my mental health all that much before I got sick. It was more of a stressful motivator to achieve, grounded in my fear-based, negative thinking. With the help of my therapist, I'm learning to evaluate my life based on those gray areas, recognizing that success is relative and also dependent on a number of factors that I have no control over.

In addition to interrupting and replacing the negative thoughts of the Inner Critic, the Worrier, and the All-or-Nothing thinker, here are a few more helpful ways to focus on the positive:

- Surround yourself with positive people—people who see the proverbial glass as half full, not half empty. Positive people help you see the bright side of a given situation and will stop you when you stray to the dark side. It's best to stay away from people who only see the negative or who put you down or belittle you in any way.
- Don't play the victim because you have Lupus. Yes, it's an awful and unpredictable disease, but you do have some control over how you react to it. You have the choice to see yourself as someone living a full life with Lupus or someone who is suffering with Lupus.
- Pay attention to how you describe your situation to others. What you say reveals how you think. For example, instead of saying, "I'm so sick of this stupid Lupus making my chest hurt so much," you should rephrase it with, "I'm looking for

new ways to deal with how and why Lupus creates pain in my chest." The latter statement opens you up the possibility of a positive outcome; whereas, the first statement is merely a negative complaint.

- List at least one thing you're grateful for every day. It helps you find the positive in your life each day no matter what you're going through at the time.

- Read positive quotes and affirmations that apply to your situation. For example, if you're anxious or fearful, find quotes that help you calm down as you replace the negative with the positive.

- Make a written list of your most common negative thoughts, and come up with alternative positive thoughts. Make a habit of reading your list often.

- Create a positive mantra to get you through. For example, "I'm glad I'm here. I'm glad you're here. I care about you. I know that I know." This is the positive mantra that I learned from Dorothy Sarnoff's book, *Never Be Nervous Again*. This book helped me overcome my fear of public speaking.[51] It contains positive statements that addresses each fear associated with public speaking. Your mantra should be a series of short sentences that counter the negative thoughts. Repeating them during your meditation ritual is an effective way to apply this concept.

Now that you understand the negative thoughts and how they affect you, you're better equipped to focus on the positive. Remember you control your thoughts and your mind. Practicing the habit of interrupting negative thoughts and replacing them with positive thoughts, in a short period of time, will lead you to gain an awareness of how much good there already is in your life, and it will attract more good to you as you make your mind more receptive to the positive.

Manage Your Stress Response

"Stress is the trash of modern life—we all generate it but if you don't dispose of it properly, it will pile up and overtake your life."

~Terri Guillemets

Manage your stress response. Notice I didn't say *control* your stress response or *reduce* your stress response because those usually aren't possible. Unfortunately, stress will always be in our lives in one form or another. There will always be situations that cause us alarm, making us choose between fleeing the situation or staying to fight it out. This fight or flight response—as it's referred to—was beneficial to our survival during prehistoric days, when we lived under constant threat of death by animal predators. Unfortunately, this physiological and psychological stress response that was designed to be protective in our prehistoric lives is now a detriment to our modern lives. It causes feelings of panic, helplessness, overload, and overreaction to situations that are not life threatening. Once exposed to a perceived threat, the stress takes over our bodies and minds—sometimes for short periods, until we can recover from the situation. But sometimes, the stress can be chronic and continue over many days and weeks. It can rob us of sleep, happiness, and can be associated with many illnesses, such as heart disease, gastrointestinal problems, obesity, to name a few.

When you have Lupus, even the slightest bit of stress can be a major trigger for flares and emergency episodes of illness. So, it's even more important for us to learn how to manage our responses to stressful situations. It may seem that this will take a lot of effort when you don't have much energy in the first place. But the effort you put in now will help change how you respond to stress mentally and thus have a positive effective physically. So, when you're in the throes of stress—feeling overwhelmed, overloaded, and overreactive—here's what to do first:

- Take a five-minute conscious-breathing break. Go someplace quiet or close your door. Close your eyes and breathe slowly. Pay attention to the air going into and out of your lungs. Breathe in through your nose, and breathe out through your mouth. This gives the adrenaline that flooded your system in response to stress time to level out, and it gives your mind a break to think more clearly and rationally. Notice how your body is reacting. Is your heart racing? Is your breathing fast and shallow? Are you sweating? Focus on slowing down your heart rate and breathing to calm yourself down. Do this for at least five minutes.

- Turn on soothing music. Create a "stress-free zone" playlist for times like these.

Once things have calmed down, take the time to incorporate the following stress prevention and management measures into your life:

- *Remove all stressors that you can control.* For example, broadcast news, both TV and radio, creates a stress response in me. I feel my heart rate increase and my anxiety take off. So, I don't watch or listen to the news. (I know this is terrible for someone who studied journalism.) I stay informed by scanning headlines online and signing up for weather alerts and emergency announcements with my local municipalities and broadcasters.
- *Remember, you don't have to respond the way everyone else does to stress.* Stress reactions are often based on contagion behaviors. Choose to think for yourself and see the situation differently.
- *Explore relaxation techniques.* Autogenic training, progressive neuromuscular relaxation, and guided meditation are very popular and effective (more on this in Chapter 10). Many of these come in the form of audio recordings on CD, Internet MP3 files, or as part of an app on your phone. Portable and accessible, these can be routinely incorporated into your daily schedule.
- *Avoid stress-based eating and drinking.* These almost always involve sugar cravings. Sweets and even alcohol only make the stress response that much worse in the end.
- *Get and stay organized.* Certain areas of your life with Lupus must be in order, to make stress more manageable—your home, your schedule, and your medical records, at the very least.

- *Learn and apply the mindfulness-based stress reduction (MBSR) techniques when time permits.* Introduced to me by my therapist, MBSR was developed by Dr. Jon Kabat-Zinn whose book, Full Catastrophe Living, gives instructions and details for applying the techniques in your life. For me, this has been a lifesaver.

Knowing that you are equipped to handle whatever happens in life goes a long way in helping you manage stress and keeping your Lupus mind healthy.

Forgive and Release
"Forgive and release. Do not allow hurts to burrow within."

~Unknown

Living with Lupus all these years, I have had my share of emotional hurts, anger, and resentments—from my friends and family, who by their actions show me that they don't always understand what it means to live in chronic pain; to my former employer, who refused to talk with me after yet another hospitalization that caused more absences from work; to my doctors, who have lost patience with me for one reason or another; to my own son, who at times has to take a break from communicating with me because Lupus and all its glory are just too much for him to take. It's even too much for me to take some times. I've even gotten angry at Lupus and at myself for somehow "getting" it.

All this hurt, anger, and resentment, though, hasn't been helpful at all in managing the disease. In fact, it's been a detriment to my mental and physical health because I've spent too much time stewing about it all.

My decision to live a beautiful life with Lupus meant that I had to let go of all this emotional pain. It meant that I had to learn to forgive. Forgive those who hurt me and forgive myself and my failing body.

Forgiveness is one of those concepts that is easy to understand to a degree, but difficult to actually accomplish. So, let's break it down:

Forgiveness means to decide to let go of feelings of resentment and/or vengeance toward people who have hurt or harmed you—regardless of whether or not you think they deserve that forgiveness.[52]

So, knowing what it means to forgive is one thing, but how do you forgive? Thankfully, I discovered that forgiveness is actually a learnable skill according to two experts in the field of psychology. First, Dr. Fred Luskin in his book, *Forgive for Good*, says that forgiveness is a simple two-step process—grieve and let go. He says it's as simple as making a choice to do so.

I also found an article in the September 2009 issue of *Psychology Today* where Dr. Ryan Howes outlines his "Four Elements of Forgiveness": 1) express your emotion about the incident; 2) understand the possible reasons for the offense; 3) rebuild trust and safety, if possible; and 4) release. Dr. Howes says that you must cycle through the first three elements until you feel comfortable moving on to the element of release and letting go.

As I see it, these two processes for forgiving are one in the same. The first three elements of Dr. Howes' process could be looked at as grieving, which is the first step of Dr. Luskin's model. Both doctors agree that the element of release, the last step in both models, is the key to reaping the benefits of forgiveness—not for those you're trying to forgive, but more so for you.

To illustrate how I've been able to apply this to my life, let's look at how I forgave my son for pulling away when I needed his support:

- *Express My Emotion.* I spent time sorting through why I felt so hurt by my son's avoidance of me. Then, I called him to discuss it. I told him that it seems that he was being cold and unloving.
- *Understand His Reasons.* Once I explained my feelings, my son told me how overwhelmed he was by my illness and that of my sister, who was just diagnosed with breast cancer at the time. He explained how he just needed a break from all the bad news. He said he was afraid of losing me and couldn't bear the thought anymore. So gaining an understanding of his point of view showed me that his actions were actually rooted in love.
- *Rebuild Trust and Safety.* I needed to get reassurance from my son that he wouldn't handle his distress this way. It wasn't good for either of us. So he agreed that he would text or send

an e-mail explaining when he needed a break. I felt reassured, and he felt off-the-hook, knowing that this way, he wouldn't hurt me.

- *Release and Let Go.* This is where I decided and promised not to hold a grudge against him; and where I decided not to dwell or ruminate on what happened.

Because I went through this process, I was able to forgive the action and release from it.

I understand that it's not always possible to work through your forgiveness steps with the person who hurt you. You can, however, still work through the steps to forgive them on your own. It might take a bit longer. Dr. Howes says that if you can't stop thinking about the offense, then you need to cycle through the first three elements again until you can truly release and let go. If you're still having trouble letting go, consider that maybe you don't want to let go of your "powerful position of victim,"[53] where you might be reaping some unidentified advantage of holding onto the grudge.

The benefits of going through the process of forgiving and releasing, you:

- Take yourself out of angry mode, which we know has the same detrimental effects as stress on your heart rate and blood pressure.[54]
- Take the burden off your already compromised immune system by removing the anxiety that weakens it.
- Create an environment for better sleep, reducing anxiety and depression.
- Cultivate healthier relationships by repairing any hurts.
- Understand that forgiveness is a process that takes time.
- Feel less pain because endorphins are no longer suppressed by your anger, anxiety, and/or depression.[55]
- See forgiveness as beneficial to you, not just the person who hurt you.
- See the silver lining in the situation because you learned something about yourself and others.

Learn About Lupus

This might sound a bit obvious, but how many of us really know and understand this disease that we have? We know it's a chronic, autoimmune disease that causes our body to attack its own healthy cells. And by now, you've read all that I've written about it in this book (and probably many other books as well). So what else is there to know?

Well, it's important to make a regular habit of remaining abreast of what's going on in the world of Lupus. Not just the emotions of its impact on your life—although that's important—but also information about how others are dealing with it and the latest research on potential treatments and therapies that may be helpful to you.

I've always operated with the motto that knowledge is power. It holds true for Lupus especially because it's incurable and its unpredictable nature often makes you feel powerless. Get some of your power back by learning all you can. Specifically, you should:

- Subscribe to the newsletters of the major non-profit organizations dedicated to spreading awareness of the disease.
- Subscribe to helpful, interesting blogs and websites on the disease that resonate with you, such as my two websites—*www.lupusdiary.com* and *www.liveabeautifullifewithlupus.com*.
- Join a Lupus support group, either online or in your local community.
- Ask your rheumatologist or internist about any news that s/he may have recently learned about Lupus.

By keeping your ears and eyes open to what's going on in the world of Lupus, you empower yourself to:

- See that you're not alone and that others are living and thriving in spite of the disease.
- Learn helpful tips and new ideas on coping and making healthy lifestyle changes.
- Give yourself options and alternatives when faced with decisions about treatment.
- Have an educated perspective on the disease.

Connect with Your Doctor

Based on research, there's an extreme gap between how doctors understand the impact of Lupus on our lives and how we as patients experience Lupus.

The reasons, according to an online global survey of Lupus doctors and patients published in *News Medical Magazine*,[56] have to do with how we express our concerns. Of the 200 patients who participated in the study:

- 60 percent say they have difficulty describing their symptoms to doctors.
- 77 percent say they only discuss the symptoms that annoy them most.
- 61 percent say they minimize symptoms to their physicians.

The majority of the participating physicians agreed all around with those statistics. But the biggest discrepancy is in how doctors see the effects of Lupus on the daily lives of their patients. While patients reported experiencing a large number of Lupus symptoms daily, the doctors think that patients only experience Lupus symptoms a few times a month.

This gap can only be narrowed by changing how we, as patients, view our interactions with our doctors. Minimizing and downplaying our symptoms and their severity, or not thinking that certain symptoms warrant discussing with our doctors, only adds to the problem.

So what can we as patients do to communicate better with our doctors?

- *Prepare for your doctor visits ahead of time.* 1) Make a list your concerns and symptoms, no matter how insignificant they may seem; 2) use your *Lupus Diary* (in Chapter 11) to make a list of any and all changes in your health since your last visit, including diet, medications, lifestyle, thoughts, and feelings; 3) make a list of questions you may have; and 4) list all of the medications that you currently take. I've created a *Doctor Visit* form that I use for this purpose. Download a free copy at:
  www.liveabeautifullifewithlupus.com/doctorvisitform/
- *Take a friend or family member with you.* Sometimes going to the doctor can be overwhelming. Having an advocate with you

will help you stay focused on your questions and help you get clarification on the information and instructions the doctor gives you.

- *Ask for the doctor's instructions.* Many times we just nod and affirm that we hear and understand what the doctor is advising or instructing us to do before our next appointment; but then we leave and can't remember a word s/he says. How many times has that happened to you? Either take along a pen and paper to write down the instructions; or ask the doctor to write them for you; or have your doctor e-mail you the instructions. You could also ask permission to record the appointment on your smartphone.
- *Ask for the doctor's email address.* Doctors are now often accessible by e-mail for questions about your situation. It saves them time and keeps you from having to wait for your next appointment to ask a question.
- *Make sure you share all reports, tests, and laboratory results with your doctor.* As I mentioned in Chapter 4, I have 10 doctors who treat me for Lupus-related issues. My internist and rheumatologist are the overseers of my treatment. When I see a different specialist or spend time in the hospital, I always ask for copies of their reports to give to my internist and rheumatologist. This keeps them abreast of everything that goes on, giving them a complete picture of how Lupus is affecting me from the perspective of other medical doctors, not just my descriptions.

For more specific issues, such as medical tests, treatment options, medications, and prevention, consider these questions to ask specifically:[57]

Questions About Medical Tests
- What will the test tell us?
- What does it involve?
- How should I get ready?
- Will insurance cover it? If not, how much will it cost?
- Are there any dangers or side effects?
- How and when will I find out the results? May I get a copy?

Questions About Your Diagnosis

- What may have caused this condition?
- How long will it last? Is it permanent?
- How is this condition treated or managed?
- How will it affect me?
- What might be the long-term effects?
- How can I learn more?

Questions About Treatment Options

- What are my treatment choices?
- What are the risks and benefits?
- Ask yourself—which treatment is best for me, given my values and circumstances?

Questions About Medications

- When will it start working?
- What are common side effects?
- Will I need a refill? How do I arrange that?
- Should I take it with food? What time of day should I take it?
- Should I avoid anything while taking it?
- What if I miss a dose?

Questions About Prevention

- What can I do to prevent a health problem from developing or getting worse?
- How will changing my habits help?
- Are there any risks to making this change?
- Are there support groups or community services that might help me?

Track Your Lupus Mind with the Lupus Diary

Following the link and instructions in Chapter 11, use the Lupus Diary to track what's happening with your mind and emotional health and the affect Lupus is having on it. Specifically, how your current symptoms, flares, and other episodes are affecting your mood and mindset. Also track your successes and or challenges with the rituals and habits to strengthen the Lupus mind, as recommended in this chapter.

Chapter 10:
Habits and Rituals to Nurture the Lupus Spirit

"We are not human beings having a spiritual experience. We are spiritual beings having a human experience."

~Pierre Teilhard de Chardin

With a soothed Lupus body and a calm Lupus mind, the path to empower and nurture the Lupus spirit is easier to navigate.

The goal here is to reconnect with something larger than your physical and mental self. There is documented evidence to show that having a spiritual connection has a positive effect on our health and well-being.

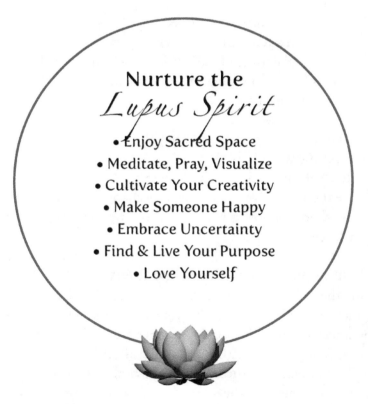

Figure 8: Habits and Rituals to Nurture the Lupus Spirit

While it's different for everyone, as discussed in Chapter 2, spirituality gives meaning and context to our lives, serves a role in our personal value system, and enables us to find comfort and hope in difficult situations. Our spirituality helps us accept the ups and downs of life as a part of a greater purpose. We can learn to nurture that spiritual connection on a regular basis by following the habits and rituals shown in Figure 8.

Enjoy Sacred Space

A sacred space is a place of reflection that you create to help you connect with your spiritual self. It can be as small or as large as you like, as long as it's peaceful, calm, and dedicated to drawing you inward. It's a drama-free zone, where everything you see, hear, smell, and touch sets the mood for spiritual reflection. This sacred space serves to remind you that no matter what's happening with your Lupus body and mind, you can always nurture your Lupus spirit by connecting to the divine place within you.

I have had different sacred spaces in my homes over the years. When raising my son alone, before the Lupus diagnosis, my sacred space was my bedroom in our tiny condo in Washington, DC, where I could lie in bed or sit in my favorite chair to take in the beautiful soothing colors of sage green and warm beige that countered the hustle and bustle outside my window. Once I moved to a larger home out West and remarried, I dedicated the guest room as my sacred space. The view of the mountains from the window is the calming focal point. I added a small open bookcase with scented candles, a few plants, and, for my achy body, a futon that's very comfortable whether it's upright as a sofa or flat as a bed. Whatever or wherever you choose for your sacred space, make sure it sets the mood for connecting with your healing by rejuvenating that connection to spirit.

Spending time in your sacred space helps your Lupus spirit by:
- Giving you respite from the pain and other physical difficulties of your Lupus body.
- Taking you out of your mental space.
- Helping you incorporate spirituality in your daily life.

- Serving as a source of creative inspiration (more about that in the *"Cultivate Creativity"* ritual).
- Giving you a place to practice additional spiritual rituals and habits.

Here are a few steps to help you create your sacred space:

1. *Discover what "sacred" means to you.* The word sacred can have very different meanings for everyone. For some, it means anything that is "highly valued, important, and deserving of respect."[58] For others, it means anything that is holy and revered in a religious sense. I'm sure for many, it's some combination of both. For me, sacred means divine, peaceful, and inspirational.

2. *Choose a place at your home to dedicate as a sacred space.* My sacred spaces have been as large as a guest bedroom and as small as a dedicated corner in a tiny condo. Look around your home and think about where you're often drawn to when you have down time. Examples include: a space near your favorite window; a sectioned-off place in a quiet room; a place on the floor with pillows to support you; in your bedroom or bathroom; outside in your garden; even within a large closet.

3. *Bring sacred elements into your sacred space.* Elements that inspire and enhance your spiritual connection, such as scented candles or incense; plants and flowers; beautiful fabrics as curtains, a blanket, or table cloth; small art sculptures; art paintings, posters, and/or postcards; divine or religious symbols; soft music; books of quotes and wisdom. The sights, sounds, smells, and touch of inspiration and peace.

Now that you have a sacred space to go to, simply be there with it at first, enjoying the peace and tranquility it brings. Then, as you read about more habits and rituals for the Lupus spirit in this section, choose which ones make sense for you and incorporate them into your sacred space. Make it a regular habit to go there every day or as often as possible to nourish your Lupus spirit, and remember you're divinely connected.

Meditate, Pray, Visualize

"The quieter you become, the more you can hear."

~Baba Ram Dass

I know that's a loaded concept for many. The idea of meditating actually used to stress me out a bit because I thought I had to transform myself into some sort of Hindu guru, sitting in a crossed-leg position. With my joint and muscle pain, that's not even possible.

Thankfully, I realized that meditation is simply defined as spending time in quiet thought and reflection when the mind is clear and the body relaxed. Those more versed in the practice use it for relaxation, for healing, for religious purposes, and/or to reach a heightened level of spiritual awareness.[59]

To get started with meditation, get into the mindset of eliminating all physical and emotional distractions. Wear comfortable clothing, and go to your sacred space or some other quiet place where you can relax in a comfortable position in a chair, on a floor cushion, or on a bed. Then begin quieting yourself, creating, as best you can, a mental state that enables you to access your subconscious mind. Then, practice the type of meditation that feels most comfortable to you. Types of meditation include:

- *Mindfulness meditation,* where you sit quietly focusing on your breathing and becoming more in tune with and aware of what's going on within your body, mind, and spirit without judgment. This is considered a very healing type of meditation because it helps you focus on the present moment and not on what has happened in the past or what could happen in the future.
- *Mantra meditation,* where you softly repeat a sound, sentence, or phrase that has a positive personal meaning to you. Aloud or in your mind, repeat your mantra in a gentle rhythm for at least five minutes. Some use meditation/prayer beads to keep track of mantra repetitions.
- *Visualization meditation,* where you close your eyes and envision a place that gives you peace, experiencing virtually all that

place has to offer—the sights, sounds, fragrances, feelings, and sensations. It's also where you envision your specific healing goals for your Lupus body and mind. Visualize your body becoming healthier and with less pain. Envision yourself living, breathing, and experiencing life in this way.

- *Breathing meditation*, where you practice breathing from your diaphragm. Start by finding a place to sit or lie down in a comfortable position; then, place your overlapped hands on your belly button. Close your eyes, and inhale as slowly and as deeply as you can, filling air into your belly region, and feeling your hands move as your belly expands and contracts. This type of meditation can be a challenge for those of us with chronic pleuritic chest pain. If this is your situation, try not breathing so deeply, or if it's still too much, simply focus on breathing normally in a comfortable position.

- *Prayer meditation*, where you connect with God or the divine being you believe in. That connection can be through praying silently or simply being with and feeling the divine presence that you recognize in worship or spiritual practice. Many people practice prayer meditation on their knees or in some other form of bodily reverence.

- *Guided meditation*, where you allow someone else to guide you through your meditation. This is often in the form of a recording, with or without background music, but can also be done in person with a meditation guide in the room with you. This is one of the easiest ways to begin a meditation practice for those of us having trouble beginning on our own. Forms of this guided meditation include autogenic training, body scan, progressive relaxation, or goal-based guided meditation for dealing with specific issues. (See the Resources section on page 103.)

Cultivate Your Creativity

"The artist prays by creating."

~Flannery O'Connor

Creativity is something brought to life "from one's own thoughts and imagination"[60]—something new and unique to you and your experience. It could be a beautiful thing that you make or a new idea or new way of thinking that you never considered before.

I see creativity as your personal expression of your spiritual self—the divine within you made manifest in your visual arts, music, cooking, dance, writings, flower arranging, scrapbooking, hobbies, new solutions to old problems, etc. Anything that you create from your own inspiration.

You'll find that this habit of nurturing your creativity is a natural extension and result of using your sacred space and practicing your choice of meditation. I often find myself inspired to get out my watercolors to paint abstracts of the colors that represent my spirit, just after meditating. It becomes an amazing visual representation of my spiritual connection at that moment in time. The joy I receive both in the doing and in the result is immeasurable.

So, to cultivate your creativity, here are a few guidelines to remember and consider as you begin to nurture this side of your spiritual self:

- Think about what inspires you—what sparks that creative energy in you. Maybe it's something that you once loved doing but haven't done since you were a child, or maybe it's something that you've always wanted to try.
- Set aside a time of day or week to be imaginative and creative.
- Feed your creativity actively by taking a course or watching instructional videos on YouTube or DVDs.
- Keep it simple and play, allowing your creativity to flow without judgment.
- Don't try to be perfect.
- Don't compare your creativity to anyone else's. Your creative pursuits are uniquely yours, reflecting your divine spirit.
- Listen to your intuition, not your conscious mind.

- Don't despair if your Lupus body affects your creativity. Recall my story in Chapter 6, where my pain affected my Lupus body so much that I could no longer practice what previously gave me joy—photography and calligraphy; but the pain led me to a new way to cultivate my creativity with watercolors, and I love it. Flowing with the changes caused by the pain of Lupus allowed me to discover something new about myself and my spirit.

Make Someone Happy

"No one is useless in this world who lightens the burden of it for anyone else."

~Charles Dickens

Up to this point, the rituals and habits I've described in this *Live a Beautiful Life with Lupus* framework focus on taking care of and protecting you so that you create an environment that strengthens, heals, and nurtures your body, mind, and spirit. So, why add the habit of making someone else happy? Well, this habit, like all the others, meets the criteria—albeit in a counter-intuitive way.

It doesn't seem logical to take the time to make someone happy when you're working so hard to take care of yourself. But, studies have shown that even the smallest acts of kindness reap health and spiritual benefits for the one doing the giving.[61] Specifically, making someone happy gives us:

- Enhanced feelings of joy and vigor.
- A reduced sense of isolation because we're connecting with others in need.
- A greater sense of self-worth and optimism.
- Decreased feelings of helplessness.
- Less awareness of our own problems when focusing on others' happiness.
- A stronger sense of purpose from being appreciated.
- A longer life—studies show that the act of giving reduces mortality rates by 40 percent.[62]

So, thankfully, those of us with Lupus don't have to spend count-less hours volunteering at a physically or emotionally draining venue. If your case of Lupus permits that, then by all means, do it. But for those of us dealing with ongoing fatigue and pain, that brand of kind-ness just isn't possible. We can, however, make someone happy with the smallest of acts, such as:

- Surprising a friend or family member with an unexpected phone call just to say hello and to listen to what's going on in their lives.
- Handwriting a note or card to send to someone you know who is having a hard time.
- Complimenting a complete stranger when you're out at the doctor or running errands.
- Donating online to a cause you believe in, even if it's just a small amount. Every little bit helps.
- Showing gratitude by saying thank you in a card or in person to those who are part of your Lupus journey—your doctors, nurses, physical therapist, or anyone who helps make your life with Lupus a little easier to bear.
- Patiently holding the door or elevator for someone who might not be able to run for it.
- Sending an e-mail to a friend.
- Sharing your wisdom and know-how with someone who might need it.
- Paying for the meal or drink for the person behind you in line.

These are just a few of the ways you can make someone happy even during the times when Lupus limits your life to bed rest and doctor appointments. When you think of ways to make others happy, you'll begin to feel your own spirits lift.

By spiritually rising above your own limitations to help someone else, you receive so much more than you give. As the old saying goes, it is better to give than receive—and that's especially true when you have Lupus.

Embrace Uncertainty

"Have patience with everything that remains unsolved in your heart....
Live in the questions now."

~Rainer Maria Rilke

To live with Lupus is to live with uncertainty. You live under the shadows of not knowing when or why a flare or major health episode will happen with your heart, lungs, brain or kidneys. The fearful thinking like—'Who knows what awful thing will happen?' and 'Oh my word, what can we do?'—prevails.

If we allow ourselves to go there—that place of all terrifying, paralyzing fear of what might happen—we're allowing Lupus to control our lives. The repercussions of this are wasted time and a life of helplessness, fear, and anxiety. On the other extreme, if we live in denial of the realities of the seriousness of the disease—in order to cope—we aren't equipped or prepared to deal when Lupus strikes. Finding the balance between the extremes of our fear of the unknown and living in denial is the goal of embracing uncertainty. It's when you face the reality of the situation, consider all possible outcomes—bad and good—and decide that you're prepared to handle either. You trust that you'll be okay, either way.

This is where the spiritual component comes in. When you can't see how things may work out, trust that God or your divine connection will know and see you through. Transcend above what your mind can comprehend in the situation, and you'll experience a peace like no other. Ever wonder why some people can smile and be happy even during the most scary and uncertain moments? Those are the people who have learned to embrace the uncertainty.

So, how do you embrace uncertainty? Here's what I've learned:

- *Face your fears.* Examine exactly what you're afraid of and why. This might sound and feel a bit ridiculous at first. *Of course, it's Lupus that scares us.* But *what* about Lupus scares you? Are you afraid that it will keep you from earning a living to support your family? That it will keep you from spending time with the people you love? That you won't be able to pay your hospital bills? That you will die? That you'll be confined to a wheelchair or bed?

- *Combat fearful thoughts with rational replacement thoughts.* An exercise that I completed with my psychotherapist is based on the book by David D. Burns, M.D. called *Feeling Good, the New Mood Therapy.* It goes like this: Take out a sheet of paper, and divide it into two columns. Label the left column with the heading, "My Current Fearful Thoughts"; and label the right column with the heading, "More Rational Replacements." Write out a list of all your fears of Lupus on the left side; then, for each one, consider ways you can counter those fears with more rational replacement thoughts, solutions, or acceptance when the situation is beyond your control. Here's one of my exercises:

My Current Fearful Thoughts	More Rational Replacements
Lupus will make me a burden to my husband.	My husband told me he loves me and wants to help and will be there for me no matter what. I choose to believe this.
I'll never find a way to deal with all this pain because my pain medications make me too drowsy to function and they don't always work.	After asking my rheumatologist about other ways to deal with the pain, she prescribed acupuncture and massage as alternatives to my pain meds.
I won't be able to afford all the doctor bills.	I will only work with doctors who participate in my health insurance plan.
Lupus will kill me, and I'm too young to die.	Most people with Lupus live long and normal lives, as long as they see their doctors regularly and take their medications as prescribed. Sure, some people die from Lupus, but that is beyond my control.
Lupus pain will confine me to my wheelchair permanently.	A wheelchair is a tool to enable me to do what I cannot do without it. So, it actually helps to free me, not confine me.
Lupus will put me in the hospital AGAIN. I can't take the thought of lying in a hospital bed with no control, dependent on others.	If I do have to stay in the hospital again, it's because my doctors care about me and want to take care of me. The hospital is a place to help me, not to harm me.

From this exercise,[63] I discovered that everyone one of my fearful thoughts could actually be countered with more rational thinking.

- *Understand that Certainty is an Illusion, Anyway.* When we realize that life sometimes blindsides us with the unexpected—no matter how well we plan—we see that we really don't have much control after all. You realize that all we do have is this moment in time, not what happened yesterday or what will happen tomorrow. Living with Lupus in the present moment enables you to manage your worry and fear about the unknown and be grateful for what you do have.

- *Let Go of Attachments to a Particular Outcome.* Sometimes Lupus makes us give up things in our lives that we once thought we couldn't live without. Take your stressful job, for example. You think you have to hold onto it for one reason or another because without it you won't have the outcome of living a certain lifestyle, for example. But, by doing so, you're detrimentally exposing yourself to stress, which is known to be a major trigger for flares. If you look at the job as something you can (and maybe should) live without, you open yourself to the possibilities of other outcomes—maybe something better. Maybe it's another job or a part-time job that meets your financial obligations while enabling you to better manage your health.   In my own life, my job and my accomplishments defined me. I worked so hard to get to my position, but one day, out of the blue, I was too sick to go on working at that pace. My health was failing, and I wound up in the hospital with the pulmonary embolism. Thinking I had no choice, I tried to go back to my old stress-filled job, which only made things worse. Once I realized that my health was so much more important than my attachment to the outcome of money and security, I released from it. Sure, I was faced with the scary uncertainty of not knowing how I was going to pay my bills and my son's tuition. But, as it turned out, releasing was the best thing I could have done. My son's school, knowing of my sudden illness, waived his tuition for that semester, which was unheard of and certainly unexpected. Then, my doctor reminded me that I could apply for disability, something so obvious that I didn't even consider. I was approved quickly and no longer had the financial worry. By letting go of my attachment to my job, I opened up the possibility for receiving more good than I could have imagined.

- *Approach Uncertainty with Wonder and Curiosity.* After this experience with releasing from my job and the perceived outcome that it was my only means of financial security, I began to see that uncertainty is really an opportunity to step back and see what good might be out there. I began approaching the uncertainty of other areas of my life with a bit of curiosity as to how others handled their issues and how good might possibly result from what I was going through at the time.

- *Practice Centering.* During those times when the uncertainty and doubt are all-encompassing and sudden—as during a medical emergency—choose to be centered.[64] Being centered is a meditative state, where you liken your position to being under the eye of the storm. Have you ever been in a hurricane? Or have you seen photographs of hurricanes from space? With storminess brewing around from all sides, under the eye of the storm, all is calm. No winds, no rain. Just blue sky and peace. As your storm passes, try mentally to stay in a centered, meditative place, likened to being under the eye of the storm, until you're able to assess the situation and apply the elements of embracing uncertainty that I mentioned.

Find and Live Your Purpose
"The purpose of life is a life of purpose."

~Ralph Waldo Emerson

Another way to nurture your spirit is to understand your purpose in this life—what God has put you on the earth to do, to experience, to learn, and to understand. Many of us, have never known what that purpose is. Or, just as we were honing in on it, Lupus strikes and takes the wind out of our sails. By practicing the habits and rituals for the Lupus body, mind, and spirit in this book, we give ourselves the best chance to awaken to the possibilities of experiencing more in this life—more of who we are and why we're here, more that keeps us alive, gives us hope and meaning.

Amazingly, some people seem to be born knowing what they're meant to do and be in life. My son, for example, started singing as soon as he learned to talk. As a toddler, he demanded that everyone watch and listen as he sang in the family room after Sunday dinner. His a cappella renditions were full of joyful, innocent expressiveness that could only come from the heart. He sang all the time, everywhere. He shared his beautiful voice throughout his elementary, middle, and high school years, and he graduated from college with a bachelor's degree in music. Now as a young adult, he gets paid to do the thing he loves. He understood early on—without much effort—his gift and continues to share it.

If only it were that easy for all of us. My experience has been the total opposite from that of my son. As a child, I bounced from one pursuit to another—art, sports, sewing, writing—enjoying them all, but never focused on any one area. I started college majoring in architecture, but ended up with a degree in business management. In my early 20s, I began working a full-time job in government finance, and I only stayed with it because it paid the bills and provided the health insurance that I needed.

The job was so stressful and unfulfilling that I found myself longing for a change. This led to my starting my own varied part-time businesses, ranging from a wedding gown dressmaker to freelance editor to personal trainer. I returned to college at the age of 38 to earn a master's degree in journalism, which led to teaching part-time as an adjunct faculty member.

No one could ever accuse me of not exploring the possibilities of other career options, even with the increasing challenges of recurring illness. In fact, the down times and absences from work with Lupus flares and episodes gave me time to reflect on what I wanted to do most and what I would regret not trying if for some reason time ran out. I also questioned why I continued endeavors that gave me no satisfaction at all. In this way, Lupus has been a blessing, reminding me that life is too short to waste time not living the way we believe we're supposed to.

After one of my most life-threatening flares a few years ago, I took a hard look back on all my starts and stops in my various pursuits at living my purpose. They were all so different, but I knew there must be a common thread among them that fulfilled and inspired me.

Then it hit me: I found that in each of those pursuits, I happily and naturally empowered people to transform themselves and their lives in some way. I helped transform brides for their big day; I helped writers express themselves more clearly; I helped my personal training clients transform their bodies; I helped my students transform their writing skills. Even during my years in the world of government finance, I found myself mentoring young women who sought career advice. My innate desire to help somehow found a way to manifest no matter how I lived and worked.

To capture and distill this revelation, I wrote my Life Purpose sentence. (Some call it your mission statement, but that sounds a bit too corporate for me.) Here's mine:

"To help people see and understand that with practice and awareness, they can free themselves to change, improve, and live a beautiful life in spite of anything that appears to hold them back."

For the record, throughout the years, I took plenty of personality tests, lifestyle assessments, and self-help quizzes. While they were helpful and surely played a role in my development, I found that the best way to approach understanding and living your life purpose is to take advantage of quiet times to work through these steps:

1. Reflect on the moments you've felt most fulfilled in life. Do not censor yourself; just allow the memories flow.
2. Determine the common threads of those times of fulfillment.
3. Use those common threads to develop your Life Purpose sentence (not paragraph). Write it out as succinctly as possible, distilling it to the very core. Note that this is not set in stone, and it can evolve over time as you develop clarity about how you want to live.
4. List out your assets—that is, your gifts, talents, skills, and abilities.

5. Ask yourself if there's a way that your assets can become the basis for living your purpose—be it as your method of earning a living full-time or as a part-time endeavor that ultimately leads you to full-time.
6. Address your fears and doubts with the exercise in the *"Embrace Uncertainty"* habit.

Once you see the wonderful possibilities arise out of the answers to these questions, your body, mind, and spirit will swell with the inspiration to make it happen in your life. You will find the courage to step out on faith to begin truly living. It may not be right away, but soon enough you'll be in the right place at the right time with the right people supporting you in your life's work.

Love Yourself

The very idea of love—being in love, falling in love, falling out of love, desperately dealing with unrequited love—can be both the bane and the ultimate blessing of the human experience. There's romantic love. There's love you have for pets and friends. There's the type of instant, unconditional love we feel for our children when we become parents. Love comes in many forms and for many reasons, but they all represent our deepest forms of vulnerability—where we dare to allow someone to be so close to us emotionally and physically that we're willing to risk our lives to avoid the pain of losing them.

From the outside world, the love we have for others is seen as admirable, a trait that only a few lucky among us are fortunate to experience. It's magical, elusive, and longed for. But what about when we think of loving ourselves? Do we feel the same level of deep affection and longing? To love yourself—*you*, with all your faults, flaws, and humanness—doesn't come naturally for most of us. Couple that with the cultural and societal influences that portray self-love as selfish and narcissistic without really understanding what is truly meant by loving yourself.

Having been passed down throughout the ages, across cultures and religions, the idea of self-love is actually considered to be among the highest of spiritual principles. We were created in love by the God or higher power of the universe who loves us. Sacred texts from

Jesus, Buddha, and others guide us to love our neighbors as we love ourselves. Many see this as a creed for a life of service to our fellow humans. Some go as far as to sacrifice self in order to make that "love thou neighbor" concept a reality.

I'm not sure, however, that we ever really, honestly, consider the "as thyself" part of that spiritual principle. My honest answer is that it has been the most difficult habit for me to implement even though I know it is most important to incorporate in my life with Lupus.

Before I began practicing the habits and rituals in my *Live a Beautiful Life with Lupus* framework, the disease had me living in what I referred to in Chapter 7 as the Lupus Disconnect. This is where my body, mind, and spirit were so consumed with Lupus that there was no opportunity for holistic healing to take place across the three dimensions of my being. In this state, I found that I wasn't very loving or compassionate with my own body, mind, and spirit. They were failing me, and I was angry. I found myself literally thinking about how much I hated myself for getting the disease. I put myself down in the most unlovable, abusive ways. And it took its toll on me, just as living in an abusive relationship takes its toll on the abused. But, I, myself, was both the abused and abuser. A very strange way to live, and certainly not a way to garner beauty in one's life.

Thankfully, as I began to understand more about this disease, develop this framework, and practice its habits and rituals, I was empowered to see myself as lovable—worthy of commitment, affection, and respect. As I worked to soothe my Lupus body, I began to accept its limitations. As I worked to strengthen my Lupus mind, I began to clearly understand my role in managing my emotional responses and in setting relationship boundaries. And, as I worked to nurture my Lupus spirit, I began to fully accept my uniqueness as a person thriving with an incurable disease. This process of inner bonding led to a deep level of love and compassion for *me*—Olivia Davenport.

To begin your process of practicing the habits and rituals of loving yourself, keep these ideas in mind:

- *Self-love is not just self-care.* It's more than pampering yourself at the spa or going on a shopping spree. Those are fleeting experiences that don't lead to any lasting feelings of self-love.

- *Self-love is unconditional self-acceptance.* You have been diagnosed with Lupus, which in no way makes you unlovable.
- *Self-love is self-respect.* This means respect for your ability to survive, to live with and embrace uncertainty, to get back up when Lupus knocks you down. You're worthy of your own admiration and esteem.
- *Self-love is having a positive self image.* When you see someone you love, you have warm and loving thoughts of that person. You see them in a positive light, even with all their short-comings. You don't put them down. Try doing this for yourself. Look in the mirror and love the person you see in that same way.
- *Self-love must be nurtured.* When babies are born, they rely on nurturing and bonding in order to grow and thrive. To satisfy the child's needs, it's natural for us as parents or caretakers to step in and fulfill that role of nurturer. Think of yourself as a child that you love. Nurture yourself. Start a process of inner bonding to understand what you need to grow and thrive as someone living with Lupus.
- *Self-love is self-compassion and understanding.* Rather than seeing yourself as less than because you have Lupus, see the situation as an opportunity to extend compassion—that feeling of wanting to help someone who is sick, hungry, or in trouble—to yourself. When we step outside of our old view of ourselves, we can see ourselves with compassion. We can see a person who deserves to be understood and loved.

Taking the time to practice the habits and rituals of the *Live a Beautiful Life with Lupus* framework is one way you are demonstrating and practicing self-love. You, yourself, are worthy of the time and attention it takes to do so.

To more deeply explore this habit of self-love, I've compiled the following list of action steps, inspired by the writings of self-love experts, such as author Louise Hay and psychologist Dr. Kristen Neff:

- On a sheet of paper, start the process of writing down what you love about yourself. If at first you're not comfortable with this exercise, it's okay. Keep at it, and treat it as an ongoing method of capturing your "loveableness." Read the list often and refer to it when you're having a bad day.

- When you have a medical episode or a Lupus flare, take time to write yourself a nurturing letter—as you would write to a friend who's going through a hard time. What would you tell that friend with love and compassion in your words?

- Prepare a statement or mantra to repeat to yourself, with the goal of reading it aloud while looking in the mirror or implementing it during your meditation rituals. To write your personal self-love mantra, consider an area that you have put yourself down, then write a statement to shed a different, more positive and loving slant on it. For example, I used to beat myself up for being what I called "an overthinker." With the help of my therapist, I came up with a more self-loving mantra to address it. So instead of putting myself down as overthinking everything, my therapist and I reframed it this way:

"I have a fine analytical mind that has served me well. I will cherish it, and I will use it without shame."

You can come up with as many or as few self-love mantras as you would like as long as your words help you to see your value and loveableness.

With practice, you'll begin to see that the habit of self-love will become more and more a natural part of who you are. You'll realize an increasing power to transform what was once self-loathing because of Lupus to self-love because of Lupus. It's all in your perspective.

Track Your Lupus Spirit with the Lupus Diary

Use the *Lupus Diary* (see full description and link to your free copy in Chapter 11) to track what you're learning about your spiritual connection. Specifically, how your current symptoms, flares, and other episodes are affecting how you see your spiritual self in this life. Also write about your successes and or challenges with the rituals and habits to nurture the Lupus spirit, as recommended in this chapter.

Chapter II:
The Lupus Diary—Holistically Track Your Life with Lupus

"Each new day is a blank page in the diary of your life."

~Douglas Pagels

It's widely accepted that the unpredictable nature of Lupus makes it imperative to keep track of how the disease is affecting our lives—for our doctors and for ourselves. Doctors need to know what our symptoms are, whether medications are effective, and how Lupus is impacting our quality of life. We, as patients, need to pay more attention to and gain a better awareness of how our actions are helping or hurting our health, which habits and rituals are working and which are not.

Like dieters and allergy sufferers are encourage to keep a food diary, Lupus patients should be encouraged to keep a diary—a daily record of how we are coping and living with Lupus. Unfortunately, the practical reality is that Lupus patients think they are too busy being sick and managing the disease to take time to track it all. But before dismissing the idea or trying and failing to keep up, consider these very positive health benefits of keeping a daily record of your health with Lupus:[65] [66]

• *A Way to Know Thyself.* Your daily writings will help you to gain a better understanding of who you are, how you think, and what makes you happy. You'll be better able to identify and eliminate the people and situations that do not support you.

• *A Way to Plan.* By recounting the day's events and experiences, you can plan what you need to do to improve the situation in the future. A Greater Sense of Well-Being. Knowing that you're keeping a record of daily life, you're not allowing Lupus to control you. You're more comfortable and confident in your ability to handle any situation.

• *A Way to Close the Gap in Our Doctor's Understanding of the Disease.* As mentioned in the "Connect with Your Doctor" habit (see Chapter 9), a high percentage of doctors say that not only are we Lupus patients unable to clearly describe our symptoms, we also

98

tend to minimize them for some reason. As a result, many doctors just do not understand the true devastating impacts of the disease on our lives. It's up to us to change that. Keeping a daily record of our lives with Lupus gives us the detailed information we need to report back to our doctors on our progress with medications and other prescribed treatments, on new and changing symptoms, and on any other matters we feel they need to know. This can go a long way toward a more effective doctor-patient relationship.

• A *New Perspective.* By writing about your days with Lupus, you have a record to look back on when life with Lupus gets overwhelming. Your new perspective will help you know that you can overcome whatever future challenges come your way.

• A *Therapeutic Outlet.* Expressing your emotions in a diary gives you a therapeutic outlet, which will help you evaluate your perspectives and perceptions in order to feel more calm and level-headed.

With these benefits in mind, I designed the *Lupus Diary* to make it easier for us to keep a daily record that will help us gain an awareness of the effect Lupus is having on the body, mind, and spirit. The *Lupus Diary*, unlike a blank diary, is divided into three sections—body, mind, and spirit. Each section contains questions, and prompts that help you write simply and directly about your day with Lupus and your progress with the beneficial habits and rituals listed in this book.

Format

The *Lupus Diary* is a PDF document that can be filled out on your computer or printed out for completing on paper. Complete your *Lupus Diary* before going to bed at night. The process will become a ritual or habit unto itself. It can be completed in 10 minutes or less; more if you want.

In the "Lupus Body" section, you write about your physical symptoms, vague or specific, trying to articulate them as much as you can, discussing whether they're better or worse than the day before or unchanged.

The "Lupus Mind" section is where you express any cognitive symptoms, emotional, or behavioral issues and feelings that are affecting you that day—whether they are positive or negative.

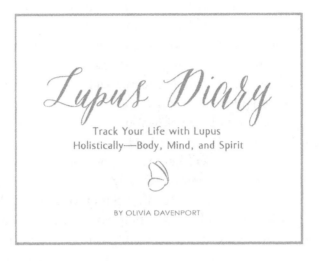

Figure 9: Cover of Lupus Diary
To download your free copy of the Lupus Diary, please visit:
www.lupusdiary.com/lupusdiary.

The "Lupus Spirit" section is where you record your pursuits at gaining inner peace and meaning beyond your physical and emotional symptoms. These include pursuits are the rituals and habits described in Chapter 10.

The *Lupus Diary* also includes a "Meals" section, where you list what you ate and how your body reacted to the food; a Thanks section, where you list at least one thing that you're grateful for that day; and a "More" section, where you're free to write and expand on your thoughts and feelings about the day.

Remember that the *Lupus Diary* is a key tool in your arsenal of living a beautiful life with Lupus. Like all of the habits and rituals of this book, the more you practice, the greater the reward—not only for you, but also for those who love you.

Chapter 12:
Are You Ready?

"The most beautiful people we have known are those who have known defeat, known suffering, known struggle, known loss, and have found their way out of those depths."

~Elisabeth Kubler-Ross

With the framework below, you can begin your journey to live a beautiful life with Lupus. I encourage you to print out a full-size version of the *Live a Beautiful Life with Lupus* framework found at: *www.liveabeautifullifewithlupus.com/framework/*

As a reminder of what you've learned in this book, hang a copy on a wall in a prominent or personal place in your home or sacred space.

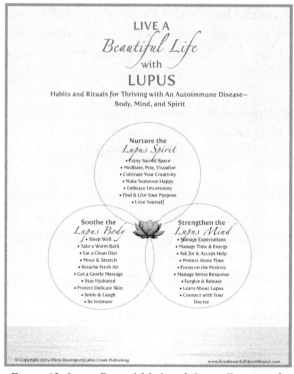

Figure 10: *Live a Beautiful Life with Lupus* Framework

Decide on the top two habits and rituals from the body, the mind, and the spirit sections that you'd like to start focusing on first. Commit to those chosen habits and rituals, incorporating them into your daily or weekly routine or schedule, as appropriate. Increase the number of habits and rituals you practice as time goes on.

Write in your *Lupus Diary* at the end of every day—just after dinner or just before bedtime, for example. Follow through on your commitment to yourself as if your life depends on it—because it does.

Living a beautiful life with Lupus is within your reach. It starts with deciding that you are more than this disease. Don't let it define you. You define it and where it resides in your life. You are not its victim, even when it blindsides you, even when you're lying in a hospital bed, fighting for your life. I know. I've been exactly there several times.

Wherever you are in life, whatever you're doing in life, simply start practicing the habits and rituals described in this book. Take baby steps if you must, remembering your commitment leads to a greater awareness, which empowers you to move forward, remembering:

"The most authentic thing about us is our capacity to create, to overcome, to endure, to transform, to love and to be greater than our suffering."

For the latest information, including up-to-date tips, news, and tools to help you live a beautiful life with Lupus, I invite you to visit my website, *www.liveabeautifullifewithlupus.com*. Also visit my *Lupus Diary* blog, *www.lupusdiary.com*, where I write in more detail about my life with Lupus and where I hold myself accountable as an example of someone who tries her best to practice what she preaches.

Resources

For additional information and assistance with the habits and rituals of the *Live a Beautiful Life with Lupus* framework, I compiled this list of websites and book titles:

Soothe the Lupus Body

National Sleep Foundation
1010 N. Glebe Road, Suite 310
Arlington, VA 22201
(703) 243-1697
www.sleepfoundation.org

"How to Pick Your Perfect Mattress"
WebMD Article by Lisa Zamosky
www.webmd.com/sleep-disorders/features/how-to-pick-your-perfect-mattress

Academy of Nutrition & Dietetics
120 South Riverside Plaza, Suite 2000
Chicago, Illinois 60606
(800) 877-1600
www.eatright.org (See "Find an Expert" link on right sidebar)

American Council on Exercise
4851 Paramount Drive
San Diego, CA 92123
(888) 825-3636
www.acefitness.org

American Physical Therapy Association
1111 North Fairfax Street
Alexandria, VA 22314
(703) 684-2782
www.apta.org (See "Find a PT" on top navigation bar)

AirNow
U.S. EPA Office of Air Quality Planning and Standards
Information Transfer Group
Mail Code E143-03
Research Triangle Park, NC 27711
www.airnow.gov

American Massage Therapy Association
500 Davis Street, Suite 900
Evanston, IL 60201
(877) 905-0577
www.amtamassage.org

USDA National Agriculture Library
Food & Nutrition Information Center
Water & Fluid Needs
www.fnic.nal.usda.gov/consumers/eating-health/water-and-fluid-needs

Centers for Disease Control and Prevention
Preventing Chronic Disease
"Behaviors and Attitudes Associated With Low Drinking Water
In-take Among US Adults, Food Attitudes and Behaviors Survey, 2007"
www.cdc.gov/pcd/issues/2013/12_0248.htm

American Academy of Dermatology
P.O. Box 4014 Schaumburg, IL 60168
(866) 503-7546
www.aad.org

Anatomy of An Illness
By Norman Cousins
New York: W. W. Norton & Company

"Laughter is the Best Medicine:
The Health Benefits of Humor and Laughter"
A HelpGuide Article by Melinda Smith, MA, and Jeanne Segal, PhD
www.helpguide.org/articles/emotional-health/laughter-is-the-best-medi-
cine.htm

"Laughter is the Best Medicine: An Interview with
Norman Cousins"
A Can. Family Physician Article by Margaret McCaffery
www.ncbi.nlm.nih.gov/pmc/articles/PMC2154152/pdf/canfam-
phys00230-0193.pdf

Strengthen the Lupus Mind

American Psychological Association
750 First Street, NE
Washington, DC 20002
(800) 374-2721
www.apa.org

American Counseling Association
6101 Stevenson Ave. Alexandria, VA 22304
(800) 347-6647
www.counseling.org

*Full Catastrophe Living: Using the Wisdom of
Your Body and Mind to Face Stress, Pain, and Illness*
By Jon-Kabat Zinn
New York: Bantam Books

The Power of Positive Thinking
By Norman Vincent Peale
New York: Prentice Hall, Inc.

Autogenic Training (MP3)
By Dr. Lynn Johnson
www.enjoylifebook.com/products-page/audio/autogenic-training/

Never Be Nervous Again
By Dorothy Sarnoff
New York: Ballantine Books

Forgive for Good: A Proven Prescription for Health and Happiness
By Dr. Fred Luskin
New York: HarperCollins

American College of Rheumatology
2200 Lake Boulevard NE
Atlanta, GA 30319
(404) 633-3777
www.rheumatology.org

Lupus Research Institute
330 Seventh Avenue, Suite 1701
New York, NY 10001
(212) 812-9881
www.lupusresearchinstitute.org

Lupus Foundation of America, Inc.
2000 L Street, NW, Suite 410
Washington, DC 20036
(202) 349-1155
www.lupus.org

Alliance for Lupus Research
28 West 44th Street, Suite 501
New York, NY 10036
(212) 218-2840
www.lupusresearch.org

American Autoimmune Diseases Association
22100 Gratiot Avenue
Eastpointe, MI 48021
(586) 776-3900
www.aarda.org

"How to Create Your Medical Records Notebook"
Article by Olivia Davenport
www.liveabeautifullifewithlupus.com/medicalrecordsnotebook/

Doctor Visit Form
PDF document by Olivia Davenport
www.liveabeautifullifewithlupus.com/doctorvisitform/

Nurture the Lupus Spirit

American Meditation Institute
60 Garner Road Averill Park, NY 12018
(800) 234-5115
www.americanmeditation.org

Center for Mindfulness in Medicine, Healthcare, and Society
University of Massachusetts Medical School
55 Lake Avenue North
Worcester, MA 01655
(508) 856-2656
www.umassmed.edu/cfm

*Inspiring Creativity: An Anthology of Powerful Insights and Practical Ideas to Guide
You to Successful Creating*
Edited by Rick Benzel
Plaza del Ray: Creativity Coaching Association Press

The Artist's Way
By Julia Cameron
New York: Penguin/Putnam Publishers

Trust the Process: An Artist's Guide to Letting Go
By Shaun McNiff
Boston: Shambhala Publications, Inc.

Feeling Good: The New Mood Therapy
By David D. Burns
New York: HarperCollins Publishers, Inc.

Additional Resources

Arthritis Foundation
1330 W. Peachtree Street, Suite 100
Atlanta, GA 30309
(404) 872-7100
www.arthritis.org

Office on Women's Health
U.S. Department of Health and Human Services
200 Independence Avenue, S.W.
Washington, DC 20201
(800) 994-9662
www.womenshealth.gov

National Heart, Lung, and Blood Institute
31 Center Drive MSC
2486 Bethesda, MD 20892
(301) 592-8573
www.nhlbi.nih.gov

National Institute of Arthritis and Musculoskeletal
  and Skin Diseases (NIAMS)
1 AMS Circle Bethesda, MD 20892
(877) 226-4267
www.niams.nih.gov

National Institute of Neurological Disorders and Stroke
P.O. Box 5801
Bethesda, MD 20824
(800) 352-9424
www.ninds.nih.gov

National Institute of Diabetes and Digestive
  and Kidney Diseases
9000 Rockville Pike
Bethesda, MD 20892
(301) 496-3583
www.niddk.nih.gov

National Institute of Allergy and Infectious Diseases
5601 Fishers Lane, MSC 9806
Bethesda, MD 20892
(866) 284-4107
www.niaid.nih.gov

About the Author

Author, blogger, and former overachiever Olivia Davenport wants to spread the news that you can live a beautiful life with Lupus. She suffered with mysterious illnesses and life-threatening episodes for over 20 years before finally getting a diagnosis of Lupus in 2012. It was then that she began a journey of research and self-discovery, to determine the habits and rituals to support her goal of not losing herself to the incurable autoimmune disease.

With her two blogs, www.liveabeautifullifewithlupus.com and www.lupusdiary.com, Olivia finds joy in sharing what she's learned with practical tools, actionable steps, and inspirational insights.

Olivia lives in Reno, Nevada with her Hubby and their odd-eyed cat, Kitty-Witty.

Index

Endnotes

[1] "Beauty." Def. 1. *Merriam-Webster.com*. Merriam Webster, n. d. Web. 10 May 2015.

[2] "Beauty." Def. 1. *Dictionary.com*. Dictionary.com, n. d. Web. 10 May 2015.

[3] Fottrell, Quentin. "Five Reasons Americans are Unhappy." *Market Watch*. Market Watch, 30 August 2014. Web. 12 May 2015.

[4] Ibid.

[5] Chan, C., Ho P.S., and Chow, E. "A Body-Mind-Spirit Model in Health: An Eastern Approach." *PubMed Health*. National Library Medicine, National Institutes of Health, 2001. Web. 17 May 2015.

[6] "Heart Facts." *Cleveland Clinic*. Cleveland Clinic, n. d. Web. 2 May 2015.

[7] "Spirit." *Merriam-Webster.com*. Merriam Webster, n. d. Web. 12 May 2015.

[8] "Spirituality." *University of Maryland Medical System*. University of Maryland Medical System, 7 May 2013. Web. 9 May 2015.

[9] "Body, Mind, Spirit: Toward a Biopsychosocial-Spiritual Model of Health." *National Center for Cultural Competence*. Georgetown University Center or Child and Human Development, n. d. Web. 22 April 2015.

[10] Anandarajah, Gowri, M.D., Hight, Ellen, M.D., M.P.H. "Spirituality and Medical Practice: Using the HOPE Questions as a Practical Tool for Spiritual Assessment." *American Family Physician*. Am. Fam. Physician, 1 January 2001. Web. 9 May 2015.

[11] "Frequently Asked Questions: Lupus." *WomensHealth.gov*. Office of Women's Health, U. S. Department of Health and Human Services. 13 June 2011. Web. 10 May 2015.

[12] "What is Inflammation?" *PubMed Health*. National Library Medicine, National Institutes of Health, 7 January 2015. Web. 12 May 2015.

[13] "Statistics on Lupus." *Lupus Foundation of America*. Lupus Foundation of America, n. d. Web. 22 April 2015.

[14] "Frequently Asked Questions: Lupus." *WomensHealth.gov*. Office of Women's Health, U. S. Department of Health and Human Services. 13 June 2011. Web. 10 May 2015.

[15] Neil Katz. "Benlysta approved: Which lupus patients will benefit?"

cbsnews.com. CBS News. 10 March 2011. Web 12 July 2015.

[16] Ibid.

[17] April Cashin-Garbutt. "Raising Lupus Awareness: An Interview with Professor Ramsey-Goldman, MD." *News Medical.* News Medical: Health News and Information, 11 May 2015. Web. 11 May 2015.

[18] "American College of Rheumatology Criteria for Classification of Systemic Lupus Erythematosus." *PubMed Health.* National Library Medicine, National Institutes of Health, n. d. Web. 12 May 2015.

[19] Ibid.

[20] "Statistics on Lupus." *Lupus Foundation of America.* Lupus Foundation of America, n. d. Web. 22 April 2015.

[21] "How Does Lupus Affect the Musculoskeletal System?" *Lupus Foundation of America.* Lupus Foundation of America, n. d. Web. 22 April 2015.

[22] "Lupus and Infections." *The Lupus Site.* Lupus Site—A Guide for Patients and Their Families, n. d. Web. 16 May 2015.

[23] "International Consensus for a Definition of Lupus Flare." *Lupus Foundation of America.* Lupus Foundation of America, 10 February 2011. Web. 12 May 2015.

[24] Kozora, E., Ellison, M.C., Waxmonsky, J.A., Wamboldt, F.S., and Patterson, T.L. "Major Life Stress, Coping Styles, and Social Support in Relation to Psychological Distress in Patients with Systemic Lupus Erythematosus." *Lupus Journal,* May 2005. Web. 12 May 2015.

[25] "Thinking, Memory, and Behavior." *LupusNY.org.* SLE Lupus Foundation, n.d. Web. 11 May 2015.

[26] Sundbom, Karrie. "Coping with Lupus." *MollysFund.org.* Molly's Fund Fighting Lupus, n.d. Web. 10 May 2015.

[27] "15 Questions – Nervous System Issues." *Lupus Foundation of America.* Lupus Foundation of America, n. d. Web. 12 June 2015.

[28] Puchalski, Christina M., M.D., M.S. "The Role of Spirituality in Healthcare." *Baylor University Medical Center Proceedings.* National Library of Medicine, National Institutes of Health, 14 October 2001. Web. 9 May 2015.

[29] Ibid.

[30] "Habit." Def. 1. *Merriam-Webster.com.* Merriam Webster, n.d. Web. 15 May 2015.

[31] "Ritual." Noun Def. 2. *Merriam-Webster.com.* Merriam Webster, n.d. Web. 15 May 2015.

[32] "Foods That Fight Inflammation." *Harvard Health Publications*. Harvard Women's Health Watch, Harvard Health Publications, Harvard Medical School, 1 July 2014. Web. 30 May 2015.

[33] "15 Questions – Strategies for Restful Sleep." *Lupus Foundation of America*. Lupus Foundation of America, n. d. Web. 19 May 2015.

[34] Ibid.

[35] "Sleep Duration Recommendations." *SleepFoundation.org*. National Sleep Foundation, n. d. Web. 15 June 2015.

[36] "How Much Sleep Do We Really Need?" *SleepFoundation.org*. National Sleep Foundation, n. d. Web. 15 June 2015.

[37] "Hot Tubs Can Land Your Heart in Hot Water." *Cleveland Clinic*. Cleveland Clinic, 3 July 2014. Web. 16 June 2015.

[38] "Things to Avoid." *The Johns Hopkins Lupus Center*. The John Hopkins Lupus Center, n. d. Web. 19 May 2015.

[39] "Stretching Exercises." *Lahey Hospital and Medical Center*. Lahey Clinic Foundation, n. d. Web. 19 May 2015.

[40] Hard, John. "Training with Lupus" *PTontheNet.org*. PT on the Net, 23 December 2005. Web. 19 May 2015.

[41] "Immerse Yourself in a Forest for Better Health." *New York State Department of Environmental Conservation*. New York State Department of Environmental Conservation, n. d. Web. 26 May 2015.

[42] McIntosh, James. "Serotonin: What is Serotonin and What Does It Do?" *Medical News Today*. Medical News Today, n. d. Web. 26 May 2015.

[43] "Enjoy Fresh Air for Better Health." *Your Standard Life*. Your Standard Life, n. d. Web. 26 May 2015.

[44] Tucker, Sheila, M.A., R.D., L.D.N. "Two-Thirds of Americans Don't Drink Enough." *BCDining.org*. Boston College Dining, n. d. Web. 26 May 2015.

[45] "Behaviors and Attitudes Associated with Low Drinking Water Intake Among US Adults,: Food Attitudes and Behaviors Survey, 2007." *Preventing Chronic Disease*. Centers for Disease Control and Prevention and the National Institutes of Health, April 11, 2013. Web. 26 May 2015.

[46] "Nutrition and Healthy Eating." *Mayo Clinic*. Mayo Clinic, 5 September 2014. Web. 27 May 2015.

[47] "Water Content of Fruits and Vegetables." *Kentucky Cooperative Extension Service*. Cooperative Extension Service, University of Kentucky,

College of Agriculture, December 1997. Web. 30 May 2015.

[48] Soong, Jennifer. "Lupus, Skin Care, and Makeup." *WebMD*. WebMD, n. d. Web. 19 May 2015.

[49] Jon Kabat Zinn. *Full Catastrophe Living: Using the Wisdom of Your Body and Mind to Face Stress, Pain, and Illness.* (New York: Bantam Books, 2013) 234.

[50] Robinson, Kara Mayer."10 Surprising Health Benefits of Sex." *WebMD*. WebMD, n. d. Web. 28 May 2015.

[51] Sarnoff, Dorothy. *Never Be Nervous Again.* (New York: Ballantine Books, 1987) 70.

[52] "What Is Forgiveness?" *Greater Good: The Science of a Meaningful Life.* Greater Good, University of California at Berkeley, n. d. Web. 20 May 2015.

[53] Howes, Ryan, Ph.D., ABPP. "Four Elements of Forgiveness." *Psychology Today.* Psychology Today, 4 September 2009. Web.

[54] "Five for 2005: Five Reasons to Forgive." *Harvard Health Publications, Volume 2, Issue 5.* Harvard Health Publications, Harvard Medical School, 15 January 2005. Web. 3 June 2015.

[55] Ibid.

[56] "Global Survey Finds Gap in Physicians' Understanding on Impact of Lupus on Patients' Lives." *News Medical.* News Medical: Health News and Information, 11 May 2015. Web. 11 May 2015.

[57] "Questions to Ask During a Medical Appointment." *National Institute on Aging.* National Institute on Aging, May 2014. Web. 23 April 2015.

[58] "Sacred." Def. 1. *Merriam-Webster.com.* Merriam Webster, n. d. Web. 10 June 2015.

[59] "Meditate." Def. 1. *Merriam-Webster.com.* Merriam Webster, n.d. Web. 31 May 2015.

[60] "Create." Def. 1. *Merriam-Webster.com.* Merriam Webster, n.d. Web. 2 June 2015.

[61] Luks, Allan. "The Healing Power of Doing Good: The Health and Spiritual Benefits of Helping Others." *MelbaBenson.com.* Melba Benson, November 2004 e-Newsletter. Web. 8 June 2015.

[62] Harris, A. H., & Thoresen, C. E. "Volunteering Is Associated with Delayed Mortality in Older People: Analysis of the Longitudinal Study of Aging." *PubMed Health.* Journal of Health Psychology, November 2005. Web. 21 May 2015.

[63] Burns, David D., M.D. *Feeling Good: The New Mood Therapy* (New York: Harper Collins Publishers, 1980) 419-423.

[64] Crum, Thomas. *The Magic of Conflict.* (New York: Touchstone, 1987) 53.

[65] "The Health Benefits of Journaling." *PsychCentral.com.* PsychCentral. com, n. d. Web. 1 June 2015. and Harvard Business Review articles. (2 separate items.)

[66] Amabile, Teresa, and Kramer, Steve. "Four Reasons to Keep a Work Diary." *HBR.org.* Harvard Business Review, 27 April 2011. Web. 1 June 2015.